Donate Your Weight

Donate Your Weight

The Stress-Free Program to Stop Dieting, Get Slim, and Help Others While Doing It

Sheri O. Zampelli

iUniverse, Inc.

New York   Lincoln   Shanghai

Donate Your Weight
The Stress-Free Program to Stop Dieting,
Get Slim, and Help Others While Doing It

iUniverse books may be ordered through booksellers or by contacting:

iUniverse
2021 Pine Lake Road, Suite 100
Lincoln, NE 68512
www.iuniverse.com
1-800-Authors (1-800-288-4677)

Because of the dynamic nature of the Internet, any Web addresses or links contained in this book may have changed since publication and may no longer be valid.

You should not undertake any diet/exercise regimen recommended in this book before consulting your personal physician. Neither the author nor the publisher shall be responsible or liable for any loss or damage allegedly arising as a consequence of your use or application of any information or suggestions contained in this book.

ISBN: 978-0-595-46536-1 (pbk)
ISBN: 978-0-595-71494-0 (cloth)
ISBN: 978-0-595-90832-5 (ebk)

Printed in the United States of America

CONTENTS

ACKNOWLEDGMENTS

Writing this book and creating the Donate Your Weight program has been a transformative experience to say the least. In some ways, this book was written against my will. Meaning that the "little" me said "No, you can't write a book like this; it's different, it's risky, it won't make sense." Then, the "big" me grabbed a pen and started writing. Nonetheless, it was only my friends and "angels" that made it possible for me to get focused, get finished and get out there. It's because of them that the book left my computer and is now available to you.

My wonderful editor, Angela Watrous seems like she can read the words between my words. She was the one who helped me see what my book was about and how I could use it to help many people worldwide. When she wasn't editing, she was coaching and encouraging. Her words and her support gave me wings and made it impossible to consider giving up.

My Master Mind partners: Cindy Schaefer, Sharareh Namjoo and Parvin Ataei provide an endless stream of inspiration and motivation for me. They show me who I really am and they believe in me and my dreams. They lovingly remind me that my limitations are all in my mind, not reality. Ray and Marty Bunch: you continually provided inspiration and support. You provided the graphics and the know-how to make my words visual.

My husband Michael Zampelli is your typical "behind the scenes" genius. He knows way more than he thinks he knows. He is my unofficial technology guru and editor. He provides the music that inspires me to soar and he brings me back down to earth when I fly a little too high. I listen, I watch and I steal. He doesn't mind and he never tries to hold me back from my true potential.

My clients, who are more alike than they are different, they all want some of the same things: peace of mind, self-love, happiness and freedom. They struggle with some of the same issues: negative self-talk, less than perfect childhoods, sensitivity and fear. They teach me and inspire me, they guide my writing and my reading choices and in the process, they help me to grow. I know that this is a mutually beneficial experience because time and again, my clients come back to tell me "thank you." It is here that I want to say: thank you. Your transformation and your gratitude give me the inspiration to keep doing what I'm doing. You let me know that I'm on the right track.

My business coaches: Casey Truffo and Jackie Nagel also helped me to see a bigger picture than I was capable of seeing for myself. All past Master Mind partners continue to live in my heart and mind and some have become life-long friends and supporters. I especially want to thank Homa Ebrahimi and Jillianne Paladino. Laura Turner, author and angel appeared in my life at just the right time. She was the answer to a prayer and we became fast-friends on the Internet. Although I have never met Laura in person, our relationship is a testimony to the fact that healing can take place across the miles.

Over the years I have led many groups, taught many classes and provided therapy to people from ages 5-72 from a wide variety of ethnic and economic backgrounds. I have worked in gang-infested neighborhoods with at-risk youth and I've provided high-cost hypnotherapy to wealthy residents of Southern California. I have worked on crisis hotlines and spent time with people in hospitals. I have heard the personal stories of thousands of people. Each one of the stories is part of the mosaic of my life. These experiences broadened my horizons, opened my mind, fueled my passion and helped me to see who I am and who I can be. Thank you to each of you for your honesty, your trust, your bravery and your determination. You rock.

Last but not least, thank you Marilyn McGraa for volunteering your time and energy to proofread this manuscript. You helped me find some of those little errors that are impossible for me to find on my own.

INTRODUCTION

FROM FOOD OBSESSION
TO FOOD FREEDOM

Donate Your Weight is a book about permanently letting go of excess weight. Millions of us have tried weight-loss plans where we decrease our calories or cut out foods that we love. But as hard as we try, and as good as our intentions are, eventually we find ourselves feeling deprived and climbing back up to our previous beginning weight and even exceeding it. Rather than another diet program that gives rules without support, this book tends to the mental and emotional aspects of your life that are ignored in traditional weight-loss programs. You will learn to identify the deep-seated habits and beliefs that are contributing to your weight problem. Most importantly, you'll learn how to build new habits that will help you release excess weight and keep it off for good.

The central message from success gurus like Tony Robbins and Wayne Dyer is that we must focus on exactly what we want to attract in life. It's a proven fact that if you want to create positive changes in life, you must keep your focus on the positive. Oprah says you need to focus on gratitude, Wayne Dyer says to "begin at the end." So why is it that with traditional diet and food plans we continually focus on the problem? We focus on losing weight (enforcing that we are overweight). We also tend to focus on what's wrong with our body—how fat we are, how uncomfortable we are, and how unattractive and awkward we feel. We call foods with fat and sugar "bad," and we label ourselves "bad" when we eat them.

Numerous authors, psychologists, and success gurus have outlined the power of beliefs and the benefits of positive self-talk and affirmations. If we focus on what we want to create in life, we will eventually create it. Some plans encourage a "tough love" approach that leaves no room for positive feelings about ourselves unless we reach our end goal. If tough love or self-incrimination worked to produce permanent weight loss, most of us would be at or near our ideal weight and large diet programs and chains would have to close down due to lack of business.

Dr. Stephen Gullo, author of *The Thin Commandments Diet: The 10 No-Fail Strategies for Permanent Weight Loss* writes, "The diet industry is leading millions of dieters to failure." He states that diets fail to take into consideration our history with food. So, for example, if you have a history of eating Kit Kats® compulsively, it might not matter at all calorie-wise if you eat a bar or two, but if you always go on a wild binge after a few Kit Kats®, it might be best to take a break from that food for a while.

Many of us have a poor body image. We see a fat reflection in the mirror no matter how much reassurance or love we get from others. Many people continue to feel fat even after they've reached their goals. In this book you'll learn how to transform your body image. This is a crucial step to permanent weight loss, because the way you view your body becomes a self-fulfilling prophecy. Thinking "I'm fat" leads to poor habits, which lead to actual weight gain. On the flipside, thinking "I love my body" leads to better self-care and a naturally healthier weight.

Inner and Outer Changes for Lasting Success

This book is more than a "weight-loss remedy" or a quick fix to get you in shape for your high school reunion. Rather, it's a way of life that begins with inner changes that ultimately impact your physical body. We need to release old painful feelings before we can maintain a healthy body weight. We need to let go of baggage like resentment, judgment, anger, fear, hurt feelings, or a broken heart. Although these are "heavy" feelings, this book can help you find creative, freeing, ceremonial, and enjoyable ways to let them go and begin the healing process. You can heal and learn to let go of negative emotional and mental baggage.

The imagination is powerful, and your body reacts strongly to what you think. If you feel unsure about the truth of this statement, consider this: what would happen if you repeated "I have a headache" to yourself for the next two hours? Instinctually, we know or fear that just thinking about a headache might eventually create one. That's exactly why it's not a good idea to continually repeat:

- I have a slow metabolism.
- I just look at food and I gain weight.
- Might as well paste it to my butt, that's where it will end up anyway.

- God, I'm fat.
- Look at these thunder thighs.

In this book, you'll discover new messages to convey to your subconscious mind that will support your ultimate success. You'll learn techniques to imagine success, because if you can imagine something first, you have a better chance of achieving it.

The mind is powerful and it pays attention to the words you use. If you eat food that you've come to believe is bad, your body will likely react in a bad way. If you feel bad or believe you are bad for eating certain foods, you are likely to engage in self-punishment or self-defeating behaviors.

The truth is, long-term, successful weight maintenance cannot be achieved by dieting. Food intake needs to be reasonable if one wants to maintain or manage their weight, but restrictive dieting just doesn't work for the long-term. As soon as you say, "I can't have _____," your interest is piqued by that exact food, and you'll think about it often until you finally eat it. If you try really hard not to think about purple cats, all you'll be able to think about are purple cats. That's why "don'ts" and "shoulds" won't work for long-term change.

This is also why so many of us overindulge in the foods we feel deprived of. We have a "feast or famine" relationship in which we fluctuate between being "good" and abstaining from the "no-no" foods and being "bad" and eating the "no-no" food in large quantities. This book will guide you in coming into a more balanced relationship with food. When you stop depriving yourself of foods you love, you can learn to eat them on occasion. It will be your choice, because you'll have taken the power away from food.

The mind has to learn to perceive change as possible and positive in order to get the body's cooperation. This book will provide you with the tools to bridge the gap. Through reading the book and engaging in the exercises, you'll learn to:

- Feel great about yourself,
- Get motivated to follow your food and exercise plan, and
- Use your mind and thoughts to your advantage.

As you read, I encourage you to keep an open mind and give each of the techniques in the book a fair and honest try—even if you've already tried some of them in the past. I often encounter folks who'll say something like, "I tried hypnosis for weight loss and it didn't work," or, "I tried affirmations and they didn't work." As I inquire and explore deeper, I find that many of these folks only tried hypnosis one time or used affirmations for a couple of days or a week. The truth is, you can't erase years and years of programming in one day or one week. That's as unrealistic as saying, "I went to the gym once and it didn't work."

While this book is full of support and proven strategies, ultimately, it's you who will make this work or not work, depending on the degree that you are willing to put in your time and energy. You'll need to commit to yourself to put what you read into practice, knowing that it will take at least thirty days before you begin to see any change. Even after thirty days, you will need to continue practicing your new skills and fine-tuning as you go. Remember, you didn't get to your current state of mind and body overnight, and it's not fair to expect yourself to make change overnight.

My Rocky Road Path to Food Freedom

I am no stranger to food and weight struggles, though many people assume I am because of the way I look. What's insidious about weight problems is that they come in all shapes and sizes (literally and figuratively). There's no predictable way to measure or weigh the amount of obsession and compulsion a person is feeling. There is no way to see or measure self-hatred.

I started out life as a naturally thin kid. Until I was twelve I was interested in many other aspects of life besides food and my weight, which I didn't think about too much. I was one of those people who seemed to be able to eat whatever I wanted with no consequence to the size of my hips, thighs, waist, or buttocks. Yet somewhere, somehow, I caught the concern. I saw pictures of models like Brooke Shields and I wanted to be thinner so I could wear tight jeans and look great. Overweight adults told me many times, "I used to be able to eat whatever I wanted when I was younger," and "You'd better watch out, if you keep it up, you'll be fat like me." I looked at them and felt petrified. I didn't want to grow up and be obese. So, though I had a slender body almost effortlessly, I began to watch what I was eating "just in case."

That was the beginning of what turned out to be an obsession with food and weight that lasted almost fifteen years and became so intense that it literally ruled my world. To complicate matters, I also began to use and abuse alcohol and marijuana as a method of escaping the turmoil in my home. I eventually became concerned that the calories from alcohol might make me fat and I didn't like the "munchies" I got when I smoked pot, so I looked for alternative ways to "numb out" or escape. By age fifteen, I was using mini-whites and over-the-counter diet aids to control my eating. I gave up drinking and used speed to control my appetite. I also smoked at least one to two packs of cigarettes a day, as another way to keep the pounds at bay. My use of drugs and cigarettes was always tied in with how they impacted my weight.

I eventually progressed in my addiction and started using hard drugs such as cocaine and heroin. Although I enjoyed the high, I was also continually making my drug choices based on how they might impact my weight. It seemed that most heroin addicts were thin, and I liked that. I didn't care if I might be killing myself in the process. I remember many days when all I ingested was a diet cola, which I paired with speed and cigarettes. I felt very successful on days like that.

Eventually drugs became their own separate problem and I stopped all alcohol and drug use when I was twenty-one. Without drugs to curtail my eating, I began to get heavier and my food addiction and body obsession became more prominent.

I joined Overeaters Anonymous, a program for self-proclaimed food addicts who just can't eat like normal people. I was a miserable failure at the program. I gained weight instead of losing and I became even *more* obsessed with food, which didn't seem possible. But I kept trying and even became the treasurer at one meeting because the commitment was supposed to help keep me faithful to my recovery from overeating. Then, on one particular night after a meeting, I felt the call of my favorite binge food: Rocky Road ice cream.

I didn't have any of my own money, but I did have money from the Overeater's Anonymous treasury in my pocket. So there I was, in line at the grocery store, buying my half-gallon of ice cream with the money from the Overeaters Anonymous treasury. Boy did I feel like a pathetic slob at that point. That was a bottom for me.

By the time I was twenty-two, I'd had bouts of bingeing, purging, and starving, along with a long list of diet failures. I was in complete emotional turmoil and literally hated myself. Then I heard a radio show that changed my life. A woman named Dr. Nancy Bonus was talking about her success in helping clients overcome food obsession and live a life free from dieting. I ended up being a client of Dr. Bonus and after experiencing success, I eventually became one of her employees. Dr. Bonus taught me about how the mind affects the body, and she was the first person who ever told me that I could eat what I wanted and lose weight at the same time.

As much as I wanted to believe her message, I figured that surely Dr. Bonus had never had a case like me. Little did she know (or so I thought) that I was capable of consuming a half gallon of Rocky Road ice cream by myself in one night. I feared I was destined to get larger and larger and more and more out of control. I literally had a vision that the paramedics would come into my apartment and have to beat my door down and resuscitate me because I had overdosed on Rocky Road ice cream.

Still, I felt I had exhausted my options, and I was ready, desperate even, to try something new. Being thin was a secondary desire; more than anything I just wanted to be sane. I wanted to go through a day where I wasn't 100 percent consumed with thinking of food, thinking of how fat I was, beating myself up for being a pig, comparing myself to anyone and everyone, and asking myself, "I wonder if I'm fatter or thinner than her?" My life revolved around my weight and my eating. Every social decision I made was ruled by whether or not there was food there, and whether or not I had something to wear that didn't make me feel too fat.

What came as an amazing surprise to me was that when Dr. Bonus told me that I could eat whatever I wanted, I almost instantly became immune to Rocky Road ice cream. In fact, I lost all interest in it. It seems that the food and the ritual of eating it were more about being bad or beating myself up than actually enjoying or craving the food itself. Being given a passport to eat what I wanted suddenly freed me from the need to see food as good or bad.

I began to learn about how powerful words are and how what I think literally creates my life. I started using affirmations and hypnosis for everything from passing my algebra test to raising my confidence and getting a new job. My life began to transform from that day forward. I began to realize that the only limitations I had in life were the ones I placed on myself. I found new, fun, freeing ways to make change. I began to unlearn old habits and replace them with new habits. I realized that I was in complete control.

As I gained this new knowledge, amazing transformations followed. I slowly (and I do mean slowly) began to like myself and my body. I began losing weight; a lot of it. My clothes were practically falling off. I went down five sizes while continuing to eat things like ice cream and hamburgers. I learned to eat more consciously and less automatically and I began to take back power and control of my life.

One of the habits I overcame was eating too quickly. As a child and young adolescent, I was a very *slooooow* eater. I remember eating one corn kernel at a time and feeling it explode in my mouth when it burst between my teeth. The adults weren't too amused by this. They told me, "Hurry up and eat, we haven't got all day" and "Stop dawdling over your food." So, eventually I guess I got fast enough and by the time I met Dr. Bonus, I was 100 percent on autopilot, almost completely tuned out from the experience. I routinely shoveled food in my mouth like an automaton. My mind was completely disconnected from my body.

When Dr. Bonus recommended eating slowly and chewing thoroughly, I *really* hated it. It seemed like forever between bites. But since I was learning about how the mind impacts the body, I realized I had to try and find a way I could learn to enjoy eating slowly. I found my solution when I realized how much of a rebel I am and decided to use my rebellion in my favor. The reason I cannot succeed at a diet is that I don't like to be told what to do. When I realized I was eating quickly because someone else told me to, I began to play a mind game. I started to say to myself something like: "Ha ha, I can eat as slow as I want and no one can stop me!" As soon as I reframed it to myself in this way, I began to revel in the joy of eating as slowly as possible. In fact, sometimes I even eat my kernels of corn one at a time, feeling them explode in my mouth as I squish them between my teeth.

To this day I love to eat slowly and I feel off-kilter when I have to rush. I'm always the last person to finish at the table, but I also have no doubt that I get more satisfaction out of my food than those who eat quickly. I began to love eating slowly once I started viewing it as my choice and my right. Not only did I start eating very slowly, I also started purposely leaving food on my plate. The rebel in me loves to see the looks of horror on the faces of people who clearly belong to the "clean plate club."

The point is: attitude is everything. You have to make change fun if you expect it to last. None of us can (or should have to) live a life of constant punishment. I've learned this lesson so well and it's made such a tremendous difference to my mental and physical health that I've made it my mission to teach it to others.

This book will teach you how to give up the struggle with weight and eating for good. You may not notice instant changes, but if you institute the concepts in this book repeatedly over a period of time you *will* experience permanent changes. You owe it to yourself to begin today to embrace steady, permanent change that will make you feel better now and next year and each year that follows. I hope you will join me on the road to permanent change. I'd love to see you there!

Donate Your Weight Program Overview

Donate Your Weight is a life-long program for health and wellness. It outlines simple daily strategies that can result in long-term weight reduction and maintenance. The Donate Your Weight program includes a comprehensive text complete with daily action plans, Seven Stress-Free Slimming Strategies, and numerous tips and techniques to overcome obstacles and roadblocks that might occur. Donate Your Weight also offers a series of hypnosis CD's and

Internet resources to help participants stop the struggle with weight and eating. Continual implementation of this program will help you form new habits and begin a new way of life.

Two powerful ways to make change permanent is to make the process fun and to include group support. In this book, you will find guidelines to form a Donate Your Weight support group or participate in a fundraising campaign. Of course, you can also choose to implement the strategies in your personal life, without a group, by reading and applying the techniques contained in this book. The Donate Your Weight program outlines time-tested and heavily researched behavior modification techniques, coupled with a fun and creative reward system that can help you to break old habits and build new ones. Use of group support and supplemental materials will help you to gain momentum with these new changes. This book also offers guidelines for large and small groups to implement the Donate Your Weight program as part of a wellness plan or team-building experience. This plan can be combined with fundraising activities to create a fun, meaningful platform for long-lasting and rewarding change.

The primary reward technique in the Donate Your Weight program is to pay yourself actual money each time you successfully complete one of the Seven Stress-Free Slimming Strategies. The goal is to make the behavior change become its own reward and to build a lifestyle around these behavior changes. As an added component of motivation, groups can decide to use the money they earned and donate it to charity.

A Donate Your Weight to Charity program offers benefits to all involved.

- Group support makes it easier to change behavior.
- Peer pressure is likely to form when individuals compete to earn the most money in their company or reach an overall donation goal.
- All the rewarded behaviors are positive, so the participant is doing something good for themselves and for others at the same time.
- An employer who offers this program is providing a positive roadmap for employees to follow. This roadmap can lead to positive change in weight, health, motivation, productivity, attitude and more.
- The techniques used in the Donate Your Weight program are time-tested and scientifically sound. They can be used to help break habits, increase sales, achieve goals, and manage troubling thoughts and emotions.
- If you choose the fundraising option, your contributions will make a difference to the charity organization you choose.
- Large donations are likely to receive positive press for the giver and the receiver and could create a wave of positive change for all involved.

Ultimately, this is a self-change program that goes beyond self-help. Those who choose to go for the gusto can create change in the world through implementing positive strategies and donating money to a worthy cause.* It's really a win-win-win situation. So, what have you got to lose? (except maybe a spare tire or some love handles).

How to Read This Book

This book contains information and resources that will outline a program for creating permanent changes in your lifestyle. The majority of benefits come not from simply reading this book but from applying the concepts outlined and utilizing the resources mentioned. Chapters 4 and 5, combined with the Success *Check*-list (Appendix II) and the Group Format (Appendix I) contain the information that will be most valuable in creating permanent, lasting lifestyle changes and stress-free slimming.

The Seven Stress-Free Slimming Strategies that are outlined in detail in chapter 4 and summarized in Appendix III are the action components of the program and will be referred to throughout the book. Chapter 5, Donate Your Weight, will outline another action component of the program and will show you how to reward your successes using real money and a reward bank, as well as explain why it's important to form or join a support group. Since the Strategies are referred to throughout the book, it might be most useful to take the following two steps prior to reading the book from the beginning. First, begin with a review of Appendix III so you can become familiar with the Stress-Free Slimming Strategies. Then go to Appendix II, where you will find a sample Success *Check*-list and a url you can use online to download additional copies of the list. Print a copy of the *Check*-list and keep it handy as you read the book. Once you've reviewed the Seven Strategies and printed the Success *Check*-list, return to chapter 1 and read the book from beginning to end. Once you are familiar with the Seven Stress-Free Slimming Strategies and have read through the entire book, you'll be in a better position to apply and personalize what you learn so you can create a program that works for your life.

---

*Sheri O. Zampelli, M.S., CCH or someone from the Donate Your Weight team is available for telephone conferences, private hypnosis and telephone coaching, and public speaking and media engagements. You can contact the Donate Your Weight office via e-mail at info@donateyourweight.com

PART I

UNDERSTANDING AND OVERCOMING THE OBSTACLES

CHAPTER I

EATING FOR ALL THE RIGHT REASONS

Have you ever noticed that infants will almost universally refuse to overeat? Not only that, they refuse to eat by your schedule. Infants know absolutely nothing about "breakfast time," "lunch time," or "dinner time." They eat when they're hungry and stop when they're full. It's only natural. Try to feed an infant even an ounce more than their tiny stomach will hold and you are sure to find yourself the loser of that battle every time.

Each and every one of us was born with the ability to love ourselves and others unconditionally. We were also born void of food rules regarding when to eat or how to eat. Young children don't have rigid ideas about "good food" or "bad food" and they don't judge themselves as "good" or "bad" for eating or not eating certain foods. We learned about food rules such as sanctioned mealtimes. We learned rules about finishing everything on our plate no matter how distasteful or massive the portion might be. We learned to judge foods based on their caloric and fat contents.

The truth is, most of us are not born with weight problems. Instead, we obtain our weight problems through the programming we receive from a very young age. Many of us become disconnected with the internal mechanisms that would help us to be naturally thin and healthy. We learn to ignore our bodies and eat by the clock. We learn to eat the amount someone else decides is right, even if it doesn't feel right to us. We gradually become out of touch with our body and its needs. We learn to override our body's natural signals about when to eat, what our body needs to eat to be nourished, and when to stop eating.

The conditioning continues when we head off to school and eat whatever is put in front of us, whenever it's put in front of us. At this point in our lives, eating times, food choices, and food amounts are most often dictated by others, not ourselves. When we later go on diet plan after diet plan, this conditioning to ignore our body's signals is solidified and reinforced. We come to believe that we can't make our own choices and that someone else must make them for us. As we get further away from our body's natural ability to guide us, we experience health and weight problems as a result.

Our body is designed to give us cues as to what it wants and needs in terms of nourishment. For example, a sudden craving for oranges or citrus fruit might be your body's way of asking for some Vitamin C, but if you're on a low-carb diet that prohibits citrus fruit, you might decide to override or ignore this craving. When you do, you have fallen prey to what's called "Diet Mentality." Part of Diet Mentality is that "they" know better. This approach doesn't allow for responding to or respecting your body's unique needs. In order to come back to your body's natural cues, it helps to first identify the distorted beliefs that serve as a barrier between your mind and your body.

Myths and Realities of Eating

Following is a list of myths and realities related to eating. Many of us are eating for reasons that have nothing whatsoever to do with nourishing or feeding our body. This list can help heighten your awareness about the myths that have been driving your eating habits. Use these new awarenesses to strengthen your commitment to cease eating on autopilot and begin eating consciously and in a way that honors you and your body. As you decide to respect your own body and its individual needs, you will slowly begin to notice changes in your eating and eventually your weight.

Eating Myth	Eating Reality
You should finish everything on your plate; there are children starving in China, Europe, Africa, etc.	You can eat and eat and eat. You can finish everything on your plate from now until eternity and all that you'll accomplish is getting fatter and fatter. The children are still starving. You'd accomplish much more good for yourself and others if you send money to hunger relief organizations and either save your leftovers for another time or throw them away. If you want to help the environment, turn your vegetable scraps into compost. It's good for you, good for your garden, and good for the landfills!

Eating food makes me feel better. It's the cure for stress and unhappiness.	While it's true that eating does provide a temporary comfort, let's look at the whole truth. Eating food does feel good, especially if you're hungry. But if you overeat or eat when you're not hungry, your good feelings will only be fleeting. After a while, it will sink in that you overate, and you'll have a whole new set of bad feelings and a barrage of self-deprecating thoughts: "Why'd you eat so much *again*? When are you going to learn? You're such a pig" (etc.). At that point, you may go to your closet once again and see all the clothes that don't fit. Perhaps you'll get yourself so upset that you'll decide to eat again, so you'll feel "better." This vicious cycle simply isn't the route to contentment and positive self-esteem.
Food is a cure for anger (sadness, loneliness, etc.) When I eat, my anger goes away.	The anger doesn't go away. It's still there, just stuffed under a pile of food that makes you sick to your stomach. And while focusing on the sick stomach does take your mind off the originating anger temporarily, eventually you're left feeling angry over the original event that angered you *and* at yourself for overeating. After repeating this cycle many times, you start to feel defeated and ask yourself, "How could I do this to myself *again*?"
If I leave food on my plate, I didn't get my money's worth.	The food costs the same whether you eat it all or not. It will end up as "waste" whether you eat it or not. If you eat when you're not hungry, you become the garbage pail and processing plant, but you still didn't save any money. In fact, you are probably losing money because of all the new clothes you'll have to buy and all the diet plans you'll try. The only thing you'll "have to show" for the money you spent is extra pounds.

Eating Myth	Eating Reality
I'll hurt someone's feelings if I don't eat it.	You can't make anyone feel anything. If a person becomes upset it's because they choose to be upset. There are many ways to show love and appreciation toward others without having to stuff yourself with food you're not interested in.
My problem is, I just love the taste of food.	There is absolutely, positively no problem whatsoever with loving the taste of food. Taste is the difference between filet mignon and hamburger meat. It's an important part of the eating experience. But it only requires one bite to "taste" something. The problem is we are often dishonest with ourselves and actually use the "taste" alibi as a way to justify overeating. Many times when we're overeating, we shovel food in our mouth nonstop with little notice of the actual "taste."
I'm just hungry all day long.	It takes about three to five hours for your body to become truly, physically hungry. Your digestive tract is about 30 feet long when extended fully; therefore, food is probably almost always in your system. Sometimes the sensation of hunger can be triggered by smell, sight, memories, etc. Some of us are conditioned to get hungry by the clock; just like Pavlov's dogs, we salivate on cue without really checking in with our body's need. A feeling of hunger can also be produced when we don't drink enough water or we eat consistently unsatisfying, low-quality food.
Food makes you fat.	Food does not make you fat. Everyone eats food but not everyone is fat. It is the misuse of food that makes you fat. For example, skinny people are often seen eating junk food but they aren't fat. Chances are, it's because they eat a little bit here and there when they feel like it. They don't deprive themselves. Dieter's on the other hand, have a 'feast or famine' relationship with food.
I might not get food like this again.	You can choose to eat anything you want at any time. If you're at a restaurant, you can take the excess food home and eat it later, or promise yourself to visit again. Overeating takes away from the pleasure of your favorite foods.

I'm healthy because I eat lowfat/nonfat foods.	Many times the lowfat and nonfat options of processed foods are high in sugar and artificial preservatives. Also, if you choose unsatisfying or distasteful foods and force yourself to eat it because it's "good for you," you will likely feel unfulfilled and therefore do more eating later on to make up for feelings of deprivation.
If I don't eat until I'm "full," I'll have to eat again in an hour.	It takes three to five hours to become truly physically hungry after you've eaten a reasonable snack/meal. If you feel hungry an hour after a meal, you may actually be thirsty or be feeling uncomfortable feelings that you're used to avoiding by eating.

Myths and Realities of Solving Your Weight Problem

In addition to myths and realities we have regarding eating, we also hold on to myths and realities regarding our weight. The following list contains a few to be particularly aware of.

Weight Myth	Weight Reality
There's nothing I can do; I just have a slow metabolism; or "Fat runs in our family."	The mind impacts the body. Repeating phrases such as these can actually create a weight problem or cause you to remain inactive/unmotivated since there's "nothing" you can do anyway. By actively fostering the new, positive beliefs you'll learn in this book, the real truth is that there's nothing you *can't* do!
If I love my body as it is, I'll just stay fat forever.	When you love something, you give it the best and treat it with respect. Treating your body with love and respect and listening to your body will naturally lead you to a healthy weight.
I don't have time to exercise.	If you don't find time for physical exercise today, you'll have to find time for physical illness later. If you replaced the time and energy you're spending denigrating yourself and your body with time loving yourself and getting physical activity, the results will be tremendous.
I'm going to pig out tonight since I'm going on a diet tomorrow.	The "pig out" only prolongs the weight problem and reinforces "all or nothing" thinking. Small, steady change will lead to lifelong results.

The scale is the best way to see if you're doing "good" or "bad."	The scale is not an immediate or accurate measure of our progress. You cannot easily measure the strength of a new habit, but new habits are crucial to your long-term, potential success.
I don't want to follow the steps in this book, it will take too long to see results.	If you don't try something different, like this steady, loving, long-term solution, you'll likely be exactly where you are today a year from now, except with another failure (and extra weight) under your belt.
Food makes me feel better.	You can never "get enough" by filling yourself with what you don't need. If you need love, reassurance, attention, or love, all the food in the world won't fill that void.
I can't be bothered to cook. Fast food and frozen dinners are good enough for me.	High quality (unprocessed, fresh, cooked with care) food is more satisfying to your body than low-quality (processed, microwaved, prepackaged) food. The quality of the foods you eat will directly impact the way you feel physically and emotionally. Eating a steady diet of processed foods is not satisfying your body's basic needs. Therefore, you might find yourself overeating in an attempt to feel satisfied. Remember, you deserve to eat fresh and healthy meals the majority of the time.

Other Misguided Reasons for Eating

You've got to admit, we are very creative in coming up with all kinds of ideas about our food and eating habits. Here are some that don't work so well. And if you read some that seem familiar, don't despair; you're going to learn ways to deal with food and weight that allow you to create a naturally slim shape and make peace with food.

"I come from a big family; if you don't grab your portion, you'll starve."

It's one thing to "grab your portion" and take care of yourself by making sure you get enough to eat. However, what often happens in these scenarios is a competition to see who can get the most. Getting the most is quite different from getting your portion. Be cautious not to get caught in a feeding frenzy mentality. If you're the cook, prepare more than enough food to be sure that your needs are met. Take your portion—not your brother's portion or your dad's portion, only yours. Focus on what you need to be satisfied and trust that there will be more food later. A positive affirmation for this scenario might be, "Today is a new day, there's plenty of food to go around, and there will be more food later if I need it."

"But the food is *free!*"

Some of us have internalized the idea that if food is available—especially if it's free—we must eat it. Of course this is not true. As adults, we get to choose when to eat and when not to eat. We never *have* to eat food just because it's there, any more than we have to smoke a cigarette "because it's there," or drive a car "because it's there," or go swimming because "there's a pool." Eating is always a choice.

Some people and places use free food as a lure to get our attention. Others use it as a way to bring people together. Either way, there is no obligation to eat or to eat it *all*. Of course, some cultural situations make it very difficult to say "no," but even in these cases, there are ways around it.

Let's look at the words "Free Food." Is it really free? Just because it didn't cost you any money, doesn't mean it's free of cost. If you eat when you're not hungry, you pay the steep price of disrespecting yourself and your body. If you overeat or eat food you don't particularly like, you pay the price of discomfort. If you overeat repeatedly, you pay the price of feeling bad about your appearance and health, as well as the monetary price of having to buy new clothes. So whether the food is free or not, ask yourself, "Is it worth the price?"

Sam, one of my clients, found that when she was in a stressful or boring meeting that had free food she always ate it, no matter if she liked it or if she was hungry. Her attitude was, "Well, if I have to sit in this awful meeting anyway, at least I can eat the food." Over time, Sam finally concluded that this attitude was ultimately self-defeating because in the end she had to endure the meeting and feel bad about herself for going against the goals she had set for herself. Everything we do or don't do has a consequence. In moments where you're being offered free food, pause first and ask yourself, "Is it really worth it?"

"I need to eat it all before my partner/roommate/family member eats it."

This is an issue that's near and dear to my heart. I can't tell you how many times I've looked forward to eating a particular food item, only to find that the person I'm living with has eaten it first. It's very disappointing. Now, if something is important to me, I make sure to put a very clear note on it saying that this food is for me and me alone! In moments when this feels challenging, or when someone doesn't respect my request, I remind myself that in most cases I can always get that exact food again later if I want to.

"More is better."

A common attitude among people with weight problems is that "more is better." A person with a weight problem may prefer the buffet over the gourmet, at least at first. But one key to overcoming your challenges with weight is to begin thinking in terms of quality versus quantity. If you eat portions that are right for you and choose from foods that are enjoyable and healthy, you'll probably look and feel much better as a result.

Remember, the "best" bites are usually the first. Food doesn't get better with each bite you take; in fact, the food loses freshness as it sits on your plate getting cold or soggy. When we eat too much, we don't feel good.

"I'm starting a diet tomorrow, so I need to finish this off today."

This type of statement is a perfect example of why diets don't work for long-term weight control. Dieting for weight release sets up a feast-or-famine mentality and wreaks havoc on your metabolism and entire digestive system. Consider the shock, discomfort, and confusion your system goes through as you fluctuate from food binge to near starvation over and over again.

Imagine your body as a manufacturing plant, complete with conveyor belts and an assembly line. When you binge or overeat in anticipation of a diet, the conveyor belt is trying to carry two to three times more items than it's used to. It struggles to move along with the overload and does the best it can. Suddenly, one of the conveyor belts stops and the items become backlogged, piling up on top of one another and falling off the sides of the conveyor belt (In this analogy, the items that fall off are equal to stored fat. Your body cannot process the extra food because it's overloaded, so it has to sit and wait until you get the plant processing things more consistently and efficiently.)

When you go on a diet and cut down on your food intake your body is playing catch up and trying to process all the extra food that you piled in the day before. If you're diligent and stick to your diet you will eventually break even and begin to make progress in releasing weight. However, many of us don't stick to diets for very long. In fact some of us are bored by the middle of the first day on a diet and want to give up. Not only do we want to can the diet completely but we want to go out for a burger and fries! If this is the case for you, can you see how this cycle will make it very difficult for your body to help you lose or maintain your weight?

The stop/start routine of feast or famine is sure to leave you feeling fatigued and almost guarantees that fat will remain in storage because the body is too overwhelmed and depleted to process the overflow. When you learn to develop a healthy relationship with food and you eat moderately each day, your body becomes a smooth-running plant where the input is just about even with the output and everything runs smoothly. This is how you can create a lifelong pattern of permanent thinness.

Eating for All the Right Reasons

Now that we've covered all the faulty reasons and excuses for overeating, let's talk about some perfectly good reasons to eat delicious food regularly and with joy. But before I do that, I just want to clarify what I mean by "overeating." Overeating is often thought of as eating a large amount at one sitting, but overeating can include eating on automatic, eating in reaction to emotions, or eating in reaction to external pressure from others. The truth is, food is fuel for your body just like gasoline is fuel for a car. The only real reason to eat is for physical hunger. Have no fear, Donate Your Weight is not a restrictive plan. In fact, I think it's important to choose several occasions a year when you allow yourself to eat simply for the sheer joy of eating. Choose three or four days of the year where you will eat for the sheer joy of eating. Maybe you'll choose Thanksgiving, Christmas, your birthday or your vacation. If you contain your eating sprees to four times a year and go back to the Donate Your Weight plan right away for the remaining 361 days, you'll be just fine. Be sure to choose really good days like a day in Julian, California eating fresh baked apple pie or a night at a fancy restaurant with succulent crab legs dipped in butter and washed down with a glass of your favorite fine wine. Please, don't waste your overeating days on cheese balls in front of the television. You deserve better than that. You won't be perfect along the road to success but you will be perfecting success. In other words, each step you take will produce a result. Repeat the things that result in positive outcomes, eliminate the things that result in negative outcomes, and learn from the things that result in neutral outcomes. As you remain committed your success plan, you'll become more and more in tune with what works and what doesn't and you will come to realize that you have total control to choose what works and ignore what doesn't.

So back to the food is fuel analogy. Think about it, you don't put just "any" fuel in your car. For example, you wouldn't put diesel fuel in an unleaded tank. You wouldn't put low-octane fuel in a vehicle that requires high-octane fuel. Therefore, you shouldn't put just "any" fuel in your body. Take time to choose the fuel that yields the highest performance so you can remain in your best condition.

Also, think about fueling your body being similar to fueling a car. Usually, you want to get to the gas station when you're close to empty but not completely empty. That's the same way you'll want to train yourself to think about food and eating. Just like you wouldn't pull over to just any gas station because "it's there," don't eat food "just because it's there." Be conscious in all your choices. Don't be a garbage pail. Be a prince or princess. Treat your body with the utmost respect and you will feel better, look better, and act better.

CHAPTER 2

CONQUERING FATTENING MINDSETS

If you want weight-reduction success that's permanent, you'll need to identify any current counterproductive mindsets that are leading to undesirable results. Then you can begin to take steps to change these thoughts and attitudes so that you're working for your own best interests rather than working against yourself. The six mindsets most likely to throw off your body image and health—deprivation, negativity, perfectionism, impatience, fear, and protection—are covered in detail in this chapter.

Fattening Mindset #1: Deprivation

Restrictive diets set up a deprivation mentality. The attitude of deprivation includes self-denigrating thoughts like: "I don't deserve good things," "I shouldn't have too much," "I'm bad for overindulging," etc. Dieters are encouraged to feel proud of their ability to deprive themselves and feel perfect and wonderful when they are successful in doing so. The problem, besides the fact that deprivation isn't such a fun place to live from, is that most humans can't endure such torture for any length of time, setting us up to feel like failures. When we finally do "fail," we feel disgusted with ourselves and we may punish ourselves by eating even more. The deprivation attitude can include depriving oneself of other treats such as hobbies, our ideal career, travel, fashion, and fulfilling relationships, the idea being that we can't have those things until we've reached our weight goals. When this happens, sometimes food is the only treat remaining available to us, and so when we finally get some we overindulge.

If you aren't sure whether you fall prey to deprivation mentality, ask yourself if you've ever experienced some version of the following scenario: "Since I already 'blew it' by eating a brownie, I might as well eat the rest of the plate. I can always start my diet tomorrow." Sound familiar? Let's look into this more.

The basic tenets of the deprivation mentality are:

- "I don't deserve to enjoy myself,"
- "I need to be punished for going outside the lines of 'good' eating,"
- "I need to eat it while I can,"
- "I must suffer,"
- "I'm bad," and
- "I'm guilty."

The inevitable results of the deprivation mentality are:

- All or nothing thinking,
- Feast or famine eating,
- Disappointment in yourself and your life, and
- Never feeling good enough.

In order to conquer deprivation mentality, you need to begin allowing yourself to have needs and trust yourself to meet them. If change is important to you, work on the exercises in this book, find an outlet for your creativity and desires, and start allowing yourself to eat a variety of foods.

Deprivation and Powerlessness

When you eat the way someone else tells you to eat, you don't learn anything for yourself, which sets up a feeling of powerlessness. You also set yourself up for cravings. Have you noticed how anytime you go on a diet or restricted food plan that you always automatically want the very thing you're told not to have? It's as if that food gains superpowers and you obsess on it day and night. It's the first thing you want when the diet is over. Whether the off-limits food is bread, fat, sugar, or tuna, you're likely to rebel. In fact, many of us find that restrictive diets set up a need to overeat or overindulge.

If you do what you're told and follow the rules of almost any diet plan, you'll probably lose weight—at first. But eventually, you have to go back to eating "normal" food and making your own choices. Since restrictive dieting doesn't teach you how to make your own food choices and how to deal with real-life eating decisions, you are likely to feel powerless again and return to the previous bad habits that caused you to become overweight in the first place. Restrictive dieting sets up an all-or-nothing, feast-or-famine dynamic that some call yo-yo dieting.

I met a woman on Weight Watchers® who struggled for weeks to lose weight. She said she was on a plateau. I began asking her a few questions regarding what she'd been doing to discover what worked and didn't work for her. As we continued to talk, she shared her frustration: "I don't understand why I'm not losing any weight! I try so hard, I eat almost *no* bread anymore." I explained to her that she could eat bread and lose weight and encouraged her to incorporate her favorite foods into her life so she could enjoy the process more and have long-term success. As she began to open up to hope that things could be different, she confessed: "I ate nine Krispy Kreme doughnuts the other day." For reference sake, one Krispy Kreme doughnut has 5 POINTS™ and of course if you multiply 5x9, you get 45 POINTS. As you look at the table below, you'll see a perfect example of how deprivation doesn't work. Take a look:

one slice bread daily	one doughnut daily	one bagel daily
2 POINTS x 7 days = **14 points**	5 POINTS x 7 days = **35 points**	8 POINTS x 7 days = **42 points**

Whether you know anything about Weight Watchers® or not, you can see that daily bread intake (even daily doughnut intake) would have been less destructive to this woman's plan than to deprive herself and then binge. She would have been better off, and probably happier to eat a little bread daily than to scarf down nine doughnuts in one sitting. Deprivation actually makes things worse in the long run.

Behavioral psychologists have known for years that the most effective way to establish a new behavior is to reward that behavior. Punishment, on the other hand, is the least effective way to evoke change. Yet for most of us, punishment is our primary tactic for weight loss. Even those of us who know that dieting isn't a good long-term solution will still punish ourselves with all-or-nothing thinking, excessive exercise, or deprivation of certain foods. Even when we don't deprive ourselves of the food, we still punish ourselves mentally by telling ourselves, "I shouldn't have eaten that," "I'm bad," "What's wrong with me?" etc.

This book will show you a new, fun, freeing way to drop pounds and keep them off. You'll learn to develop rewards that genuinely support your long-term success. You'll also learn about shaping. Shaping is the psychological term for starting where you are and making small, steady steps to move to where you want to be. You may have also heard it called taking "baby steps." When using shaping, you should set goals small enough so that success is almost guaranteed. The more times you are able to succeed, the more motivated you will be to continue succeeding. In their book *Self-Directed Behavior*, David L. Watson and Ronald G. Tharp provide two simple rules for shaping: you can never begin too low, and the steps upward can never be too small. When you combine rewards and shaping over a long period of time, you'll gradually make permanent changes and your new behaviors will become automatic.

Goodbye Deprivation, Hello Satisfaction

One of the main reasons we overeat is that we are not getting the full satisfaction and pleasure out of eating. We think that by eating "more" we will get "more" pleasure, but that's not actually true. What is true is that some foods are more satisfying to us on more levels than others. One of the keys to moving away from feeling deprived is to seek foods that are genuinely satisfying.

Many people will agree that fresh, home-cooked foods are more satisfying on more levels than most frozen or fast food meals can ever be. A home-cooked meal is usually prepared with fresh ingredients for a small group of people. It has the very-real ingredients of love, creativity, and personal touch. As corny as it may sound, these ingredients are absolutely a part of the satisfaction we experience when we enjoy the process of eating a home-cooked meal. When someone prepares a meal for us, or even when we prepare a meal for ourselves, we feel nurtured. Underneath it all, a home-cooked meal says, "I'm worth the time and energy it takes to prepare this food."

The process of cooking can have its own pleasures. The scent of the food as it cooks is an indulgence all its own. The scent on your fingers after chopping fresh basil or garlic is a part of the experience. Watching the food, stirring it, and tasting it are all part of the experience that can increase satisfaction with food. Compare this to the ritual of taking a box out of the freezer, putting the frozen rectangle into the microwave, and eating the steaming-hot concoction out of a small, plastic container. Certainly two different experiences, with one being significantly less satisfying!

Even if you're not an experienced cook, try purchasing fresh, organic items for one meal and notice the difference between how satisfied you feel eating them as opposed to processed, manufactured foods. Fresh fruits and veggies from a farmers market taste amazing because they've often been picked the same day. Produce sold in chain grocery stores is often picked or harvested before ripeness, and it can be 3 to 7 days until it reaches the stores. The difference in satisfaction between eating fresh produce and week-old produce is tremendous.

Likewise, a handmade, gourmet sandwich from a corner bakery can often be fresher and more satisfying to the palette and olfactory glands than a sandwich from a corporate chain that uses bland ingredients with many preservatives. For true satisfaction, you want to "dine" rather than eat. Find a way to eat a wider variety of healthy, fresh, quality foods when possible. The dividends will pay off handsomely in health, satisfaction, enjoyment, and a slimmer waistline.

Savor the Experience of Eating

Another way to gain greater satisfaction out of food is to savor it by eating slowly and chewing thoroughly. Imagine eating food the same way a wine taster tastes wine. Inhale the aroma. Notice the subtleties of the scents. Can you identify any of the key ingredients by scent alone? Next, cut the food and notice the texture and firmness. Is this food chewy, crunchy, melty, silky, grainy, smooth, etc.? Notice any juices, sauces, or fillings as they ooze out. Bring the food to your mouth slowly. Notice the aroma becoming stronger. Notice any sensation of hot or cold as the food is near your mouth. As you open your mouth, notice how it prepares for the incoming bite by producing saliva. Notice your mouth's reaction when the food touches your tongue, gums, and teeth. As you chew, notice the seasonings and the temperature. Continue chewing and enjoying the food until it dissolves in your mouth. Swallow and take a pause. Ponder how much you enjoyed what you just ate and if you didn't enjoy it, *stop eating it and get something else instead!* Pause consciously and make a decision before automatically taking another bite.

Refrain from anything that resembles shoveling, cramming, stuffing or "pigging out." That's not your style! Put on the food taster hat and savor every bite. Stop before you get full. That's right … before. Remember, this is about enjoying food, feeling satisfied. Do you truly enjoy being full or stuffed? Learn to tune into that moment when the amount of food you've eaten is "just right." Then, push the food away, walk away from it, or put it away. Revel in pride as you enjoy feeling "just right" instead of feeling like a "stuffed sausage." The more you practice with this, the better you'll get. You will learn to love that "just right" feeling and overeating will become very uncomfortable and foreign to you. Remember, if you accidentally under-eat, there will always be more food later. You don't have to eat it all now and you don't have to spend hours moaning in agony as you ask yourself, "Why did I do it again? When will I learn?"

Indulge Your Senses in All Areas of Life

As long as we're talking about engaging the senses, let's not forget there are many other potential pleasures in life besides eating food. Be sure to treat yourself to non-food sensory experiences daily. You have at least five, maybe six senses: sight, touch, sound, smell, taste, and (I'll posit) intuition. How much attention are each of your senses getting? Perhaps one or more of your senses is so deprived that you're trying to compensate by overindulging the sense of taste. Remember, it's never a good idea to spoil one sense and ignore the others. It's simply a recipe for disaster. I mean, imagine if you had six kids and you ignored five of them and spoiled the remaining one senseless (pun intended)? How about six hamsters or six plants or six houses? Whatever it was, if you ignore five and overdo it with one, you're going to be in big trouble. So, let's talk about those other senses besides taste and see how you can begin to give them the love and attention they crave.

Sight

What do you look at every day? Is it pleasing? Is it stressful? Is it possible to change it? Would you feel better if you changed it? When can you start? When did you last go to an art show or slowly peruse the pages of a beautiful book or magazine? You don't have to go completely wild and rearrange your entire house or office, but little things can make a big difference in satisfying your sense of sight. How about adding a picture of something that brings you joy, a houseplant, or a piece of art. Maybe you can rearrange things so you have a nice view out the window. When your visual landscape is pleasing, you'll have less stress and therefore less need for stress-induced eating. Similarly, if your visual landscape is stressful (i.e. piles of unfinished business; worn, torn, tattered, or dirty objects), you're more likely to end up at the refrigerator or snack machine without even knowing why. Who really wants to stare in the face of an overwhelming mess day after day? Visual overload from the computer or TV can also create stress. Try to take breaks from extended stays in front of either monitor. Go for a walk or step outside and regroup from time to time.

Touch

Are you giving and receiving hugs? Have you received or given a good massage recently? Have you ever tried finger-painting, ceramics, or gardening? There are numerous ways to engage the sense of touch. Perhaps you can pet an animal or go to the fabric store and feel the texture of various fabrics. Choose some luxurious, comforting sheets, pillows, or towels for a sensory treat. You can spend time in the yard touching various plants or even the soil. Perhaps you might engage in a hands-on hobby such as crocheting or making puzzles.

Sound

What is your soundscape like? Are you hearing any pleasant sounds? Are you hearing distracting, annoying sounds? Are you taking time to listen to your favorite music? Simple adjustments such as adding a table fountain or environmental noise machine can help to create a more pleasing environment. Perhaps you can listen to your favorite music while you work or maybe even create your own music in your spare time. As much as possible, try to drown out or eliminate sounds that might be annoying or stressful.

Smell

Have you indulged your sense of smell lately? We can often transform our mood by changing the scent we are exposed to; a loved one's cologne, the smell of home-cooking, scented candles or incense, fresh flowers, the wilderness, or the aroma of a favorite restaurant are just a few scents that can soothe and uplift us. We can engage our sense of smell in numerous food and nonfood ways. Start focusing more on your sense of smell when you eat, and create an environment of soothing scents you can enjoy as a boost between meals.

Intuition

While not commonly listed as one of the senses, intuition is actually a very important sense. Unfortunately, we often don't trust our sense of intuition in the moment; instead, when something fails or doesn't go our way, we might say, "I knew something was wrong; I felt it in my gut but I didn't follow my intuition." Once you learn to accurately tune into this sense in the moment, following your intuition or "gut feeling" can save you time and energy. In order to develop your sense of intuition, you'll have to engage in a trial-and-error process: when you follow your intuition and get a favorable outcome, you'll start to develop a deeper trust in yourself. Developing this sense leads to feelings of high self-esteem.

Fattening Mindset #2: Negativity

When your focus is on negativity you regard yourself as flawed and "not good enough." Focusing on the problem leaves your mind closed to solutions. When you decide that "there's no hope and no point," you may also figure there's "nothing" you can do to change your situation—which is a completely untrue, because there is *always* something positive you can do. Yet because you believe there's nothing you can do, you do nothing and so there is no change.

When you are engaged in negative thinking, you see the proverbial glass as half-empty. You neglect to give yourself credit for any small successes, such as not feeling proud when you don't gain any weight while on your weight-loss program. You may also fail to notice any of the good things that happen, like when you lose a pound, even if your goal was to lose 5 pounds. If you're trapped in negative thinking, you may find yourself thinking thoughts like: "What's the point? It always ends up the same anyway," "I'll probably just fail again, so I'm not going to try anymore," "I'm just born to be fat, there's nothing I can do about it," or "I'm too old, and this is just the way things are."

Negative thinking can lead to feelings of depression, sadness, or cynicism, and can lead you to isolate, stuff your feelings, or simply give up. But even if your negative thinking is habitual and ingrained, you can conquer it. Begin by identifying negative thoughts for what they are, and recognize that they aren't the truth, they're just a temporary negative opinion. Acknowledge to yourself that negative and positive outcomes have at least an equal chance of coming true.

Then begin to analyze your automatic, negative thoughts. Challenge their validity with factual feedback or positive affirmations that counteract your negative self-talk. You may want to practice "cool thoughts," which are factual thoughts that you intentionally use to diffuse negative thinking. For example, a negative thought might be, "I'm a loser and a fat cow. No one would ever date me." The cool thought would be: "I'm overweight. I don't feel good about myself yet. But there are many people my size and larger who are in loving relationships right now."

Fattening Mindset #3: Perfectionism

Perfectionism and procrastination go hand in hand. Perfectionists wait for the "right" moment to get started. They want everything "just right," but sometimes you have to accept that maybe it will never be "just right" and that it's time to accept what's happening and make the best of it.

If you're engaging in perfectionist thinking, you may think you're never good enough, focusing only on flaws and always thinking things could or should be better. You may find yourself having thoughts like, "That's *all* you did?," "I guess I did okay with my eating, but I *only* exercised three times this week," "I really blew it yesterday," or "I *only* lost one pound this week, I should have lost more."

Perfectionist thinking can lead to feelings of anxiety, stress, fear, or loneliness, and may lead you to isolate or become controlling of yourself or your environment. When you suffer from perfectionism, you may also have trouble recognizing your perfectionism or understanding how the sample sentences are examples of perfectionist thinking. If you're thinking, "How could I be a perfectionist? I'm far from perfect," you very well may be a textbook perfectionist. Still, there's always hope, and you can conquer perfectionist thoughts. Begin noticing and focusing on all successes, small or large. Give yourself praise for your accomplishments, no matter how small. Believe in yourself, allow yourself to be human, and stop comparing yourself to unrealistic ideals.

Fattening Mindset #4: Impatience

Long-term, permanent weight release is not a race. If you're seeking to get slender and stay slender, you'll need to cultivate patience with yourself and the process. Currently, you probably have the attitudes, behaviors, and habits of an overweight person—which is why you're overweight. You can change your attitudes, behaviors, and habits to be those of a person with a healthy weight, but these changes don't happen overnight. It will take time to raise your awareness, institute new habits, and allow them to become an ingrained pattern. If you're impatient with yourself, you'll probably be tempted to go back on a restrictive diet that provides temporary, quick weight loss, forgetting that this approach leads to immediate weight gain after you end the diet. I'm here to remind you that quick fixes never achieve long-term affects. You can save yourself lots of heartache and discouragement by instead starting to change the habits that made you overweight in the first place. With new habits, you will eventually create a new body.

If you're looking at the situation from a place of impatience, you may be having such thoughts as, "It's never good enough," "I want to *see* results now," or "What do you mean I only lost one pound? I have been good all week, I even exercised three times."

When you're stuck in an impatient mindset, you may refuse to focus on the small changes that are happening, focusing instead only on the scale and beating yourself up for not trying harder or getting faster results. You may find it hard to stick to a long-term plan, getting impatient with yourself and wanting instant results.

Having an unchecked impatience mentality can leave us never feeling fully content or "good enough." Especially when we have a long way to go, it's incredibly painful when our impatience causes us to discount all progress and success as "no big deal," as if only the end goal is a positive result. You can conquer your impatience by learning to focus on all aspects of change and by being honest with yourself. Honestly evaluate all the years it took you to get to where you are now, and understand that it will take time to establish new habits. Remind yourself that taking this time to go slowly and establish new habits will ultimately lead to positive and lasting results.

Fattening Mindset #5: Fear

When we engage in fear-based thinking, we entertain "worst case" scenarios and build scary stories that keep us stuck. Change is a scary thing, even when it's a positive change. When we fear our own weight-loss success, we may have thoughts like, "If I lose weight I might get too much attention." "If I get thinner I won't be as strong." "If I lose weight, I'll have to buy a whole new wardrobe and I can't afford it." "I'll lose some of my friends if I get too thin." "What if I can't handle it?" "What if I lose weight, only to fail again?" "What will I do with all my time if I don't have to worry about my weight?" "What will other people think?" Our fear of failure or fear of success may lead us to sabotage our efforts, because we're afraid of the negative feelings we may have if everything does not go perfectly.

When you engage in fear-based thinking, you may feel depressed, immobilized, or "stuck," or you may isolate yourself. Fear is a very powerful emotion, but it can be conquered. Start by taking slow, steady steps toward your desired goals and know that you can handle it. Remember, change is usually slower than we'd like it to be. As you move through the process of change, it will prepare you for the end results. Talk about your fears with supportive loved ones. Most of the time what we fear is going to happen will never happen. Do you want to waste your mental energy preparing for something that will never happen? If not, try to entertain the idea that a "best case" scenario is equally possible.

Embarking on a weight-loss journey can be hard, sad, intimidating, empowering, scary, exciting, freeing, challenging, and more. Ultimately, it's up to you how you view the changes you're beginning to make. If you can begin to perceive change in a positive manner, you'll be more likely to succeed. The upcoming chapters will give you tools, techniques, strategies, and examples that can make this process enjoyable and freeing. You can learn the skills for life-long change and get off the yo-yo roller coaster for good.

Fattening Mindset #6: Protection

For some of us, extra weight feels like protection from unwanted sexual advances or feared intimacy. But there are other ways to protect ourselves, like healing past wounds and developing healthy boundaries. Our excess weight only hurts us further.

Overcoming Sexual Abuse and Rape

If you've been sexually abused or raped, your abuser may have told you that you "brought it on yourself" because you were being "sexy." Often in this case, our mind/body system deduces the following "solution": Don't be sexy and that won't happen again. Unfortunately, this approach just doesn't work (not to mention that it deprives us of experiencing a healthy sexuality and high self-esteem about our bodies). Sexual abusers carry out their act to wield power over a victim. Sexual predators do not choose a victim based on looks; instead, they choose a person who is defenseless or weaker than they are. Carrying excess weight is no guarantee that sexual abuse will come to a halt or never happen. It is *never* your fault if you're abused.

There is nothing anyone can do to 100 percent guarantee protection from abuse. Yet every day you carry weight as a form of protection, you actually harm yourself more than you help yourself. Even twenty-five to thirty extra pounds can put extra strain on your heart and increase your risk of cancer. According to a 2006 press release from the American Cancer Society, "being overweight is a risk factor for many forms of cancer, including breast cancer among post-menopausal women and colorectal cancer. It is estimated that about one-third of the 564,830 cancer deaths that are expected to occur in the United States in 2006 will be attributable to poor nutrition, physical inactivity, and being over-weight or obese. Nearly two-thirds of Americans are overweight, including 30 percent who are obese." (Source of statistics: Cancer Facts & Figures Prevention & Early Detection 2006, American Cancer Society.)

Holding on to extra weight as a form of protection leaves us feeling uncom-fortable and not as mobile or fit as we would like to be. Several women I coun-sel talk about the agony of being in a body that prevents them from even being able to tie their own shoes. Every day that we hold on to excess weight and live in an unhealthy, uncomfortable body, it's as if our abuser is physically and mentally holding us hostage. We are in a prison, though we have committed no crime.

If this sounds familiar, now is the time to free yourself from prison. Find a therapist you trust and who is well-trained and experienced in handling the abuse issues you're dealing with. Understand that you are not to blame for any abuse or unwanted sexual advances you've experienced. Find new ways to pro-tect yourself, such as a self-defense class. Join a support group where you can come to understand that you are not alone and that there is a way to heal.

Make a commitment to yourself to reclaim your power and take back your body. Release the pain and the weight, and allow your body to become a size and shape that's comfortable and healthy.

Avoiding Unwanted Sexual Attention

Even when we haven't been sexually or physically abused, many of us are taught, either through words or experience, that being in good shape will bring on unwanted sexual attention. We may notice that others flirt with us more frequently when we're thin, and this attention may awaken our own sense of our sexuality, which can feel scary if we've been told that sexual feelings are "bad," or can feel tempting if we're in a monogamous romantic relationship.

It's important to understand that all humans are sexual beings—as well as spiritual, mental, physical, and emotional beings. We (thankfully) cannot successfully rid ourselves of our sexuality, even if we carry over 100 extra pounds on our body. So rather than trying to hide what's such a natural part of yourself, embrace your sexuality. Own it and know that you are in control of how you will express it. If you don't feel in control now, you can increase your feelings of control in therapy or in a safe, supportive group of helping individuals. There are healthier and more fulfilling answers and solutions to these fears than simply carrying excess weight.

As many of us have discovered, the extra weight doesn't provide a guarantee of safety from sexual urges and advances. Many have found that they continue to receive flirtatious gestures from others even when they are overweight or obese. It's important to honor yourself and deal with the feelings and underlying fears directly. Extra weight can actually kill us slowly. Isn't it better to find new, life-enhancing ways to deal with these fears? We can learn to set boundaries and be assertive so that sexual gestures won't have as much power over our lives. We can learn to identify the signs of inappropriate behaviors, and we can sever relationships that are uncomfortable or unhealthy early on, before abuse occurs.

I once met a man who told me he was carrying an extra 50 pounds on his body because every time he got thinner, he attracted more female attention. This man had once been unfaithful to his wife during a time when he was slim. He feared that if he allowed himself to be thin again, he might have another affair. His extra 50 pounds served to protect him and protect his marriage. Although the intention was commendable, neither he nor his wife was happy about his physical condition. With therapy and support work, he was able to learn new skills to avoid unwanted attention, such as:

1. Not initiating or encouraging flirtation of a sexual nature

2. Not placing himself in situations where he would be alone with some-one of the opposite sex
3. Creating a statement in advance that he would use whenever he sensed he was in a "sticky situation" (one statement he used was, "I have to go pick up my wife so we can meet with our son's teacher")
4. Joining a support group and selecting one or more people who were willing to let him call when he needed to debrief from a situation

Numbing Painful Feelings

Excess weight can also be evidence of an attempt to numb ourselves from uncomfortable feelings or painful, unresolved memories. Some mind/body theories believe that when a person is traumatized, they store the trauma in their body. Some people even experience the sensation of being "stuck" or "frozen" after experiencing a trauma. Traumatic events include dramatic life experiences such as the death of a loved one; a car accident; sexual, physical, emotional, or verbal abuse; chronic neglect or rejection from a parent; witnessing a crime, or any number of smaller but nonetheless painful or scary incidents.

While trauma is not uncommon, the effects need not be permanent. Talk therapy can help and many body and somatic therapies are also known to help a person effectively release trauma from the body. However you attempt to release your past traumas, it is important to do so. It is believed that stress trapped in the body may actually slow down the digestive process. It is the equivalent of hair trapped in the sink drain. Until it gets unstuck, the flow of water is drastically slowed down. A person who feels frozen or stuck is likely to avoid physical activity for fear of reactivating the trauma. Handling this trauma in a safe environment will help you to get back on the road to becoming slimmer naturally. In the book, *Energy Tapping*, authors Fred Gallo and Harry Vincenzi provide the readers with excellent somatic releasing techniques for releasing trauma. Releasing trauma and feeling your emotions are major components in long-term weight loss and maintenance. See the resource section in the back of the book for information about mind/body therapies that can help you release trauma.

Feeling Solid, Stable and Secure

For some, being large feels like protection simply because being small can be associated with being weak, fragile or easy to push around. Extra weight can cause one to appear strong or powerful and can even be a valid defense mechanism for a person who feels internally weak or small. It's important to remember that there are many ways to build internal strength and as you do, it will feel safe to let the external weight go.

A thin, frail figure can be associated with fears of terminal illness. For example many people with cancer or AIDS become very emaciated prior to their death. Subconsciously one might equate a solid, hefty body with freedom from illness. However when excess weight begins to create its own set of health problems, it's important to drop the fears of being thin and embrace thoughts of health and vitality.

CHAPTER 3

STOP THE STRUGGLE WITH WEIGHT AND EATING

For so many of us, our problems with weight and eating have involved such a painful struggle for so long that we can't imagine a life without it. We can even forget that such a peaceful existence is possible. But in this chapter, I'm going to share five simple truths with you that will help you stop the struggle with weight and eating:

1. Your mind and body respond to the words you use.
2. Eating food doesn't cure anything except physical hunger.
3. Your mind and body respond to your actions.
4. Food only has the power you give it.
5. If you can envision it, you can achieve it.

Your Mind and Body Respond to the Words You Use

What you think creates how you look, plain and simple. Take the example of Daisy, who always felt like she'd look better if she lost 5 to 10 pounds. She was never really overweight until she reached her thirties. However, from the time she was sixteen years old, she always said things like, "I'd like to go swimming, but I'm too fat to wear a bathing suit," or, "What guy would want to date a fatty like me?" It took fifteen years of referring to herself as "fat" before she actually became overweight. Now she looks at her pictures from high school in astonishment and asks herself, "How could I ever have thought of myself as fat?! I looked great. I only wish I looked like that now!" Daisy's story is one that many of us can relate to, and it reminds us of how powerful our thoughts are over our perceptions and our behavior. Consider the following example of a common negative thought that leads to an unhelpful action and an undesirable result:

Original Thought	Action	Result
"I'll never lose weight."	You figure you might as well eat unhealthily and skip the gym, since you'll "never lose weight" anyway.	You not only fail to lose weight, but you continue to gain weight, thus "proving" yourself right!

Perhaps you have thoughts like, "I'm fat," "I'm too lazy to change," or "I can't deal with this." But here's the thing: just because you think something, it doesn't mean it's true. Still, when we think something is true, we search for evidence to prove it, focusing on the parts of our body we think are too big or the things we do that "prove" we'll never change. Once we have "proof," we react with more negative criticisms and judgments, or we react on a subconscious level and feel discouraged, depressed, angry, or hopeless. Eventually, we feel so fat and miserable that we decide, "What's the point?" and we reach for high-fat, high-sugar comfort foods to "feel better," or starve ourselves and wreak havoc with our metabolism, setting ourselves up for future overeating episodes. This thought/feeling/behavior interaction creates a self-fulfilling prophecy that either results in a real weight problem, as happened to Daisy, or worsens an already existing problem.

Now imagine if current research in quantum physics is true and each one of our thoughts is an electrical impulse that impacts our brain and creates neural pathways and chronic ways of thinking. Can you imagine how many millions of self-hate and unhealthy thoughts and feelings our body is processing all day? Every time you compare yourself unfavorably to others, or give your eating power over to someone else, or think negative thoughts about your body, you are sending signals to your body and your body is obeying your commands. Every time you walk past an ad of a perfect image that you'll never attain, or watch a TV show, the constant message you are reinforcing about yourself is "not good enough" and "can't measure up." Figures 3.1 and 3.2 below demonstrate how the mind can impact the body.

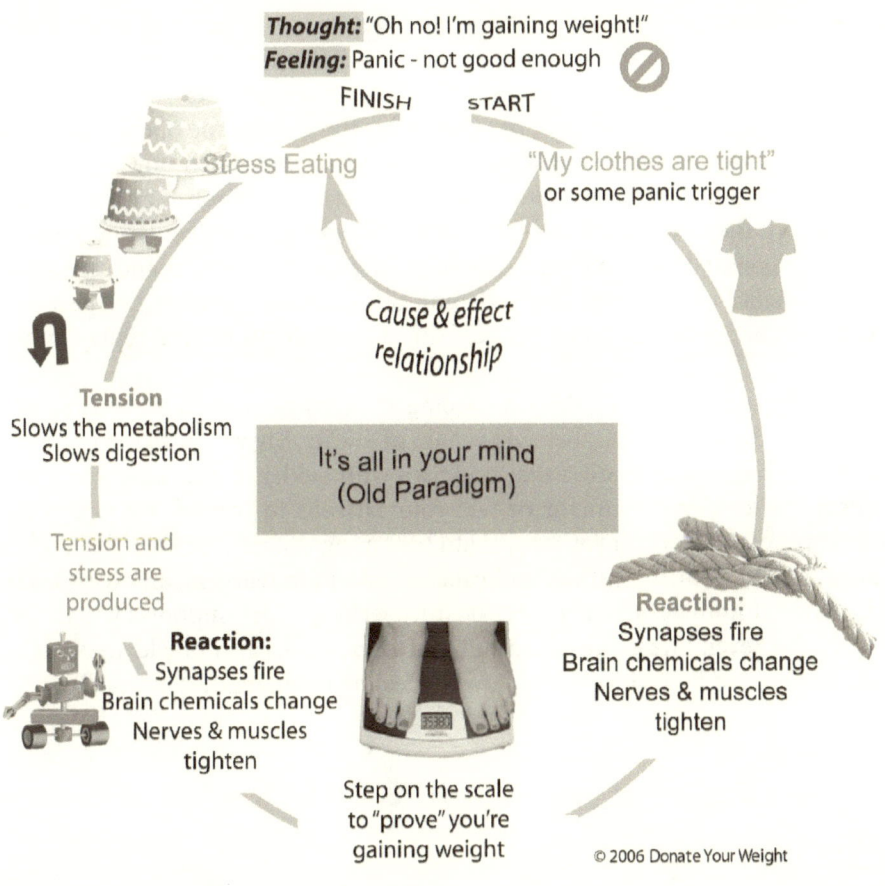

Fig. 3.1

The good news is you can actually shift your energy as you shift your thoughts. Therefore, you can literally create a different perspective of reality. It is not a right or wrong choice but should be a choice that works best for you. For example, you can choose to be grateful for legs that carry you from place to place rather than looking at your legs and seeing spider veins or cellulite. You can be happy for your arms that allow you to hug and hold and carry rather than looking at the extra flesh in your upper arms. You have a choice regarding what you focus on. Some of us are choosing to focus on what's wrong with us, what's wrong with our lives and what's wrong with our bodies and this is what makes us miserable.

I saw a young woman for 3 hypnotherapy sessions. In her first session, she expressed grief and sadness about her childhood. On the third session I helped her remember some of the playfulness and spontaneity of her youth. I helped her to reframe the experience of her past. After the session, she opened her eyes in amazement. She said "wow, I had no idea I had that much power over my thoughts." You see, she was stuck in two or three strong memories or "stories" of the past but they were nowhere near the totality of her experience. She learned in three sessions that she could choose a different perspective and therefore her experience of life would be different. She could not change her past but she could change what part of her past she chose to focus on and replay in her mind.

Let's play out a scenario, this time seeing what happens when we consciously change the thought/feeling/behavior chain of events. Say you have the thought, "I am fat" but before feeding that criticism with evidence, this time you stop, refusing to look in the mirror or feel your fat rolls to "prove" your negative thought. Instead, you tell yourself, "I am becoming thinner," or "No, that's a lie. I am actually beautiful, strong, and capable, and I am releasing all excess body fat." This naturally results in a more positive feeling, which supports you in following the Seven Stress-Free Slimming Strategies. This also breaks the potential chain of bad behaviors that follow the feeling or thought, "I am fat."

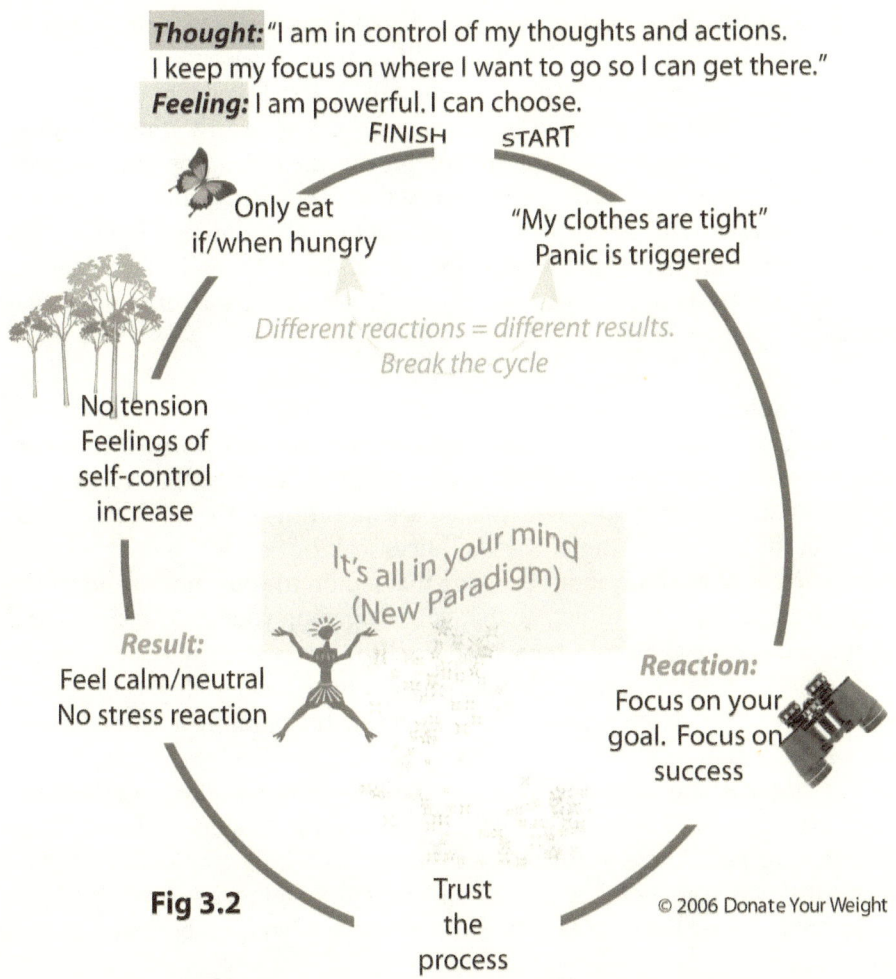

Thought: "I am in control of my thoughts and actions. I keep my focus on where I want to go so I can get there."
Feeling: I am powerful. I can choose.

FINISH   START

Only eat if/when hungry

"My clothes are tight" Panic is triggered

Different reactions = different results. Break the cycle

No tension Feelings of self-control increase

It's all in your mind (New Paradigm)

Result: Feel calm/neutral No stress reaction

Reaction: Focus on your goal. Focus on success

Fig 3.2   Trust the process   © 2006 Donate Your Weight

If you're triggered to call yourself "fat" because you are comparing yourself to someone who's thinner than you, you can choose to think statements like, "I am doing my best," and, "I claim my right to determine what is attractive by my own standards." If temporary bloating triggers the "fat" feeling, you can say, "I am temporarily bloated, but that's not the same as being fat." If after reaching your healthy goal weight (which a medical doctor can help you determine for your age, height, and body type), you still feel fat or see yourself as fat, you can state the facts by saying, "I am a healthy weight for my height and age," "I am at my goal weight," or "I'm at the size that's best for me."

Choosing these new perspectives over the old, automatic reactions will cause your body to have an entirely different reaction. You will have stopped the chain of events that triggered overeating or feelings of low self-worth or defeat in the past. Slowly but surely, you will begin to create a new reality, a more positive self-fulfilling prophecy. You'll stop falling prey to the old, automatic reactions of beating yourself up or overeating. Your setbacks will be smaller, shorter, and farther apart. Gradually, you will gain control of your mind and body so you can find a weight that's comfortable for you and stay there. It begins with a choice to say positive things to ourselves. We are all capable of making that choice.

Understanding Mind Power

The words you think and say and the associations you've formed with particular words impact your body in a very real way. To see how this works, close your eyes and imagine you've just taken a lemon out of the refrigerator and you're cutting it with a knife. See the juices leak out as you slice the lemon into quarters. Now think about bringing that lemon to your mouth and smelling its fresh, citrus scent. Imagine that you're opening your mouth slowly and then sinking your teeth into the lemon. Feel the tangy, sour juices explode in your mouth. If you imagine this scenario vividly, it's likely that your mouth will water. Your body may respond as if you are actually eating a lemon, just by imaging it.

The words we say to ourselves have a similarly powerful affect on the body. Read the following sentences slowly and with feeling. Imagine different times when you've heard these words and from whom. Notice the tremendous impact it can have on your body just thinking about the memories associated with these words. Pause between each line and notice how your body reacts:

"I'm sorry."
"I love you."
"You're stupid."
"You'll never succeed."
"You're amazing."
"You can do anything you set your mind to."

Positive words can shift your focus, calm your nerves, and evoke positive, forgiving, or loving feelings. Negative words can cause you pain and drain your vital energy and hopefulness, especially when they're coming from within. Notice how your body chemistry can actually change just from thinking words.

Imagine, then, how much more impacting words are when you hear them repeatedly. Think of the difference it would make in your life if you heard a vindictive, "I hate you!" every day versus a heartfelt, "I love you."

The Woman Who Died of an Abbreviation

The placebo response demonstrates the power of the mind over the body. It's the theory that your belief about medicine might be as important, or more important, than the medicine itself. In research studies, participants were given sugar pills but were told that the pills were a strong headache medication. Participants who took the sugar pill reported a decrease in symptoms. Some even stated that their headache completely went away. Over the years, many study participants have been cured of their illness, though the prescription they've been given is, unbeknownst to them, a thirty day supply of sugar pills. What this shows is that even when a "medication" has no medicinal value whatsoever, it can still work as long as the patient believes it will work.

In Howard Brody's book, *Placebo Response,* he shares the following story about a patient, Mrs. S who "died of an abbreviation." Mrs. S. had a non-life threatening heart valve condition called tricuspid stenosis and was in the hospital for a check up. At one point, "the senior cardiologist came into her room, accompanied by a bevy of residents, interns, and medical students ... the group talked among themselves–treating the patient as if she were an object, paying no direct attention to her, and excluding her from their conversation." The senior cardiologist told the interns, "This woman has TS"—employing an abbreviation cardiologists commonly use for "tricuspid stenosis."

When Mrs. S' primary Dr. came back to see her she was anxious, frightened, and breathing fast. "That doctor said I was going to die for sure," said Mrs. S. "He said I had T.S. I know that means 'terminal situation.' You doctors never tell us the truth straight out. You always try to hide it to soften the blow. But I know what he meant."

The Dr. tried to explain that by "TS" his senior had meant "tricuspid stenosis," not "terminal situation." Mrs. S. insisted that she "knew" the Dr. was just trying to protect her. She died later that day.

Mind Over Matter

If someone actually caused their own death because of a belief, isn't it a logical next step to think that your hateful words to your body have caused your body to become one that you're prone to hate? To see how you've created the body you have right now, answer the following questions honestly:

- What negative words do you use when you talk about your body?

- How do you describe or think about your metabolism?
- When you look in the mirror, what do you notice? What's the first thing you see?
- When you put on an item of clothing that's snug, what words do you think? How do you feel?

Considering your answers to these questions, does it seem likely that there might be a relationship between your thoughts and feelings about your body and the actual size and shape of your body? Does it make more sense to you why you are currently dissatisfied with the health and shape of your body?

What body do you think you'd have if your answers to all of those questions were positive? What if you think and say that you have an active, rapid metabolism? What if you focus on what's right about you versus what's "wrong" with you? What do you have to lose by giving positive thinking a try? (Nothing much, except your extra weight and your poor self-image!)

Athletes use the power of positive thinking all the time to enhance their performance. Imagine for a moment that you are an athlete preparing to compete in the long jump. You begin to prepare for the jump and tell yourself, "Oh man, I'm never going to make this jump. What was I thinking?" Then, bang, a gun is fired and you must now get a running start and prepare to jump. Your chances of doing your best in this event aren't very high. But if, instead, you visualize yourself making a record-breaking jump beforehand and you think to yourself, "I can do this!" your chances of success are exponentially greater.

Now, look at the scenario from a weight-loss perspective. You are overweight and you want to get into good shape. You haven't been in good shape for years. You say to yourself, "Geez, here I go on another diet. Who am I trying to fool? I'll never be able to get to my goal weight. After all, I'm older now, my metabolism isn't as fast as it used to be. I'm going to have to cut out all sugar and fat until I get rid of this fat. It'll be miserable." This may sound harsh, but this kind of negative self-talk is common among people trying to lose weight. It also almost guarantees failure.

Let's take a closer look at this process so you can better understand how it works and why it's counter-productive to your success. Imagine that you plan to lose 20 pounds, but you focus on the possibility of failure, rather than your plan for success. You start your new eating program, even though you say to yourself that you're never going to make it. You bombard yourself with self-criticisms and harshly berate yourself for your existing weight problem and for everything you eat. As a result, you begin to feel powerless. Instead of focusing on what you do have power over, such as your ability to adapt the Seven Stress-Free Slimming Strategies, you instead focus on the times you slip and don't use the Strategies. You start indulging in all-or-nothing thinking, and decide that unless you can lose 5 pounds a week, it's not worth it. To achieve this unrealistic goal, you decide that you're going to have to cut out all fat and all sugar forever. This rigid rule is impossible for you to keep to over time, so you overindulge, get discouraged, and give up on using any of the strategies in this book. You end up gaining more weight, and feeling like a terrible failure, which leads to more negative thinking and an ever-intensifying cycle of self-neglect and self-criticism.

As you can see, the way to success and satisfaction is to cultivate positive self-talk and a positive outlook about all of your endeavors. Since the mind so greatly affects the body, it's very important to be attentive of what we say to ourselves about our body and how it processes food. What you say is what you get. If you believe you are *never* going to be thin, you'll prove yourself right. If you believe you will *always* have a weight problem, you'll be right. And who wants to be right about something like that? The great thing is you can choose to believe, "My body is efficient and smart. I get better every day" and that will also come true.

Our behavior is impacted by the thoughts and images we hold about ourselves. If we think of ourselves as "weak", we won't try as hard. If we think of ourselves as powerless, we won't assert our power. By the same token, if we see ourselves as fat, ugly, old or not good enough, we will likely create a lifestyle, attitude and demeanor that makes us appear and act more fat, old, ugly and not good enough.

Don't Lose It, Donate It

While we're in the topic of the power of words, think about the words "lose," "loser," "lost," and "losing." Now, answer the following question, without ever referring to weight:

1. Name a time in your life when you were happy to lose.
2. How would you react if someone walked up to you and said, "You're a loser!?"
3. How does it feel to be lost or to lose something?
4. What do you feel after a loss?
5. Would you rather be losing or winning?

As you can see, the word "lose" and its derivations can have negative and depressing connotations. In most areas of life, losing is a sad, painful, or embarrassing feeling. When we lose something, we try to find it again. We most often hear, "I'm so sorry for your loss," not, "Congratulations on your loss!" So when we talk about "losing" weight, doesn't it make sense that on some level the mind would want to avoid "losing" and all the pain that comes along with it?

That's why I encourage you to think of an alternative language when you refer to your slimming body. Let go of your weight. Release it. Surrender it. Free yourself from it. Heck, why not *donate* it by using your weight loss to help humanity (see Chapter 5 for the full details). At least when you donate something, you feel good about it. It's final, and you don't plan to get it back. After you reach your goal you can say, "I donated my weight to charity."

The Good, the Bad, and Their Impact on Our Bodies

The words "good" and "bad" have tremendous impact on our mind/body connection. In our culture, we've misguidedly categorized foods as "good" or "bad" based on their calories, fat or carb content, their amount of sugar, and so on. In the dieting community, food is most often termed "good" if it's low-fat, low-sugar, and high fiber, and "bad" if it isn't these things.

Unfortunately, many of our favorite foods can fall into this "bad" category, and when we put ourselves on restrictive diets that demonize any particular foods, the healthy foods we're supposed to think of as "good" become our enemies.

We then call ourselves "bad" for eating less nutritious but good tasting foods, and call ourselves "good" for eating food that part of us sees as "bad." This becomes very confusing to the mind and the body. With all these mixed messages we send to ourselves, it's no wonder we don't achieve the success we desire!

Instead of all this labeling of good and bad, it's time to just see food as food. As you build a different relationship with food that's about fuel instead of about reward, you will start to notice that some foods have more nutritional value than others. That doesn't mean you can never eat foods that aren't packed with nutrition. You can simply learn to enjoy fueling your body in a healthy, more balanced, and less judgmental way.

If you're thinking, "I can never eat fast food again if I want to be slim," realize that these kinds of deprivation "never" thoughts are really counterproductive to your long-term goals. Behavioral psychologists have known for many years that if you want to successfully make permanent behavior changes, you need to focus on rewards, not punishment. In other words, you need to focus on what's good about changing and how you'll benefit, not what you'll lose or how you'll suffer. Research also shows that clear, direct, consistent communication reaps greater results than indirect, unclear, inconsistent communication—so it's important to be clear about your goals and consistent with your language so you can speak and act in a way that will help you achieve that which you truly desire. Since you want to look and feel good, focus on words and beliefs that will propel you in the direction of looking and feeling good.

It's All in the Name

Most people with weight problems have some negative associations related to the words "diet" and "exercise." Is it any wonder, considering that we've endured torturous, painful diet and exercise plans in the past, during which we've bombarded ourselves with negative thoughts and words? However, there are many definitions of the word diet. Maybe its time to change your paradigm about dieting. The New Webster's Encyclopedic Dictionary of the English Language defines diet as: "food and drink considered in terms of composition and effect on health." Well that's a wonderful definition: basically, realizing that food impacts health, and making a choice to eat food because it's good for you. Beats the heck out of my diet definition: "eating stale, boring, tasteless, preservative-filled, artificially sweetened food that gives you gas, makes you pale, makes you want to kill your family, rots your teeth and turns you into a crazed maniac who will shuffle into the kitchen like a robot and eat anything in sight at about one a.m."

How about exercise? My aunt actually calls exercise the "e word" as if it's too awful to speak out loud. What if you called it playing instead? I don't know about you but when I was a kid, riding my bike was not exercise. I lived for the times I could get on my bike and feel the wind on my face. I loved to weave in and out of the lines in the road and make my bike sway from side to side. When portable audio players became available I loved to put on my favorite cassette tape and ride my bike to the beat. The music was so motivating that I pushed myself to ride up big hills and pedal on the straightaway as fast as possible. I lived to hula-hoop, jump rope, play foursquare or handball. I was thrilled to play on the swings, the rings and the monkey bars. At the park, you couldn't stop me from throwing a Frisbee or climbing a tree. Guess what, it was all exercise. Good thing I didn't know it.

Now at age 40, I have trained myself to get back in touch with that enthusiasm. When I get to go for a bike ride, I feel like the "happiest kid on the block." For fun, I bought myself a pink beach cruiser that I ride up and down the boardwalk. I purposely wear fun clothes: a pink tee-shirt that says, "Future Celebrity" and my big pink glasses with rhinestones in them. I top it off by wearing my pink iPod. It gives me that extra attitude I need to shift my mind and have fun rather than "suffer through" the experience. It's true, attitude is everything. I have toured the same bike path with a sense of heaviness, dread and self-loathing. It was quite a different experience.

I have found music to be a key element for my motivation. Some songs are fun and have such a great beat that it makes it near impossible not to move. I choose songs that are uplifting and have a great beat so I am pumping nothing but positive energy into my personal time. If you listen to negative, problem-filled music and exercise, you will cancel out the full potential benefit of physical exercise. Your mind and body will be opposing each other because one is focused on negative and the other is trying to do something positive. A positive recharge can go a long way to help you feel happier and achieve more.

Food Doesn't Cure Anything Except Physical Hunger

Many of us have an engrained habit of using food to "cure" our anxiety, boredom, sadness, anger, loneliness, or other uncomfortable feelings. We may have even used food to push down uncomfortable positive feelings, numbing our successes and happiness, and allowing food to come between us and our relationships and dreams.

As (uncomfortably) comfortable as this habit is, the truth is that the only thing food cures is physical hunger. Using food to deal with emotional issues may prove to be a distraction, but it doesn't *solve or improve* anything, and it gives food too much power in our lives.

Eating for comfort also creates another problem: excess weight (which, of course, is an excellent distraction as well). An important step in solving your weight and eating issues is learning to eat primarily for physical hunger and to honestly assess in each moment whether or not you are eating to satisfy physical hunger or to "deal" with emotional issues.

One way to determine if you're truly, physically hungry is simply pause before eating and ask yourself: "Am I truly, physically hungry?" It takes at least three to five hours for your body to become truly, physically hungry after a reasonably sized meal. So, if it's been less than that amount of time, chew some gum or drink water. Ask yourself, "If I could have anything I wanted right now (non-food related), what would it be?" Write the answer in a journal about your feelings. Keep track of the feelings that trigger your desire to eat and see if you can nurture and honor those feelings in a different way.

You might find with consistent journaling that your hunger is not for food at all. The hunger might be triggered by boredom or impatience or stress. We might feel excited or nervous or scared and that feels like hunger. Or maybe we're eating to kill feelings or squelch desires. Many of us are living in a very restrictive box of our perceptions and don't allow ourselves to step out of these rules for fear of rejection, retaliation, abandonment, chastising or other things we've learned to fear over the years.

Fears might come packed as lies like, "I can't promote myself, I'm not as good as other people, if you knew the real me, you wouldn't love me, I just don't know what I want, or I just don't care anymore." It's important to begin identifying these nasty critters so you can kill 'em and clean 'em out of your life. They are not true and they are literally stopping you from reaching your potential.

As you identify fears, replace them with positive affirmations. As you identify emotional wants, needs and cravings, vow to find a way to feed them. Some clients find that they wrap themselves so much into their job and their family that they don't take any time for themselves. This is a real disservice to you and to those around you. Depleting yourself like that means you're giving your family a defective version of yourself. Give them your best self. You can only do that if you give to yourself first.

You may discover that your solution is as simple as a hug, a shoulder to cry on, compassion, understanding, or a good, old-fashioned pep talk. As you learn to identify what you need and you send a clear signal that you want it and deserve it, you will get it. Allow your emotions the opportunity to be acknowledged, they are there for a reason.

At first, as you learn to identify your true needs and feelings in the moment, it may still be challenging to figure out how to avoid eating when you aren't hungry. Here are four positive alternatives to "emotional snacks":

1. Chew gum,
2. Drink a glass of water with a slice of lemon, orange, or cucumber, or
3. Go for a walk.
4. Write in your journal. End on a positive note by writing at least one thing you're grateful for or listing at least one thing you love.

If all else fails and you still decide to eat, even if you're not hungry, it's really important that above all else, you *forgive yourself!* Beating yourself up doesn't do anyone any good. Instead, see if you can learn from the experience. Acknowledge all the positive changes you've made up to this point, and brainstorm at least one way you can try to do things differently next time.

If you're eating for emotional reasons on a regular basis, see if there's a new way you can deal with these emotional issues. Consider therapy or a support group, and/or the affirmations, visualizations, or self-hypnosis strategies suggested in this book. If you're running from a dream or stuffing down a passion, commit to taking time for those dreams to be fulfilled. Consider a career or life coach. Create time in your life to pursue your passion.

Your Mind and Body Respond to Your Actions

Communication is multi-faceted. It includes verbal, nonverbal, and even subconscious properties. Communication skills classes, parenting classes, sales training courses, and even dog obedience classes teach us that effective, consistent communication is the key to getting results. The most effective communication is consistent: the verbal and nonverbal match each other. However, it's rare that individuals are aware of how to communicate with themselves effectively. It seems to be a well-kept secret that communication skills which are widely used in business and interpersonal relationships can be used effectively in intrapersonal communication as well.

Changing your thinking is an important step in reducing stress, changing habits, and feeling better. However, you know the old saying: "Actions speak louder than words." The actions you take are sending messages to your body, and if your thoughts conflict with your actions, guess what wins? If you regularly say to yourself and others, "Health is my number one priority," yet your actions are knowingly unhealthy (you smoke, you don't exercise, you eat junk food), you're sending a mixed message and are therefore not as likely to get full cooperation from your mind/body system, which could otherwise be providing you with inspiration, creative ideas, and, gradually, a new way of doing things. If, alternatively, you say "Health is my number one priority," and you back it up with action, your mind and body will be in synch with each other and you're more likely to have a harmonious, seemingly effortless journey toward healthier and healthier choices.

Since this concept can be hard to conceive at first, I'm going to provide several examples of how bringing together thoughts and actions results in the greatest success, starting with the non-food example of Joanne, who went into therapy because she was unhappy with her marriage. Joanne felt like she was the one doing all the work and that her husband took her for granted. She continued to ask her husband for help but he had excuses and said she was nagging him. One day, she had the following realization in therapy: "I say, 'I need help,' but then I do everything I want done myself. I'm not consistent with what I say and what I do, so I don't end up getting the help I want." In order to back up her words with matching actions, Joanne stopped taking the trash out and let the dishes pile in the sink, since those were the jobs her husband agreed to do. She proved that she needed help by letting things go. It was very difficult to see the mess at first, but eventually she started to get the help she needed. She still has to occasionally resist the temptation to pick up after others, but she's also learned that if she doesn't do it, someone else always does. It's not a perfect system, and things don't always happen on her timetable, but she does get help, she's much less resentful, and she finally has some free time for herself so she can take better care of herself.

Gilda had a very similar experience with the importance of matching her words with her actions. She was following the techniques described in this book, including hypnosis sessions, listening to affirmation CDs, and beginning to consciously change mental habits. And she was having great success: she was wearing the smallest size she'd been in six years, and she felt less stressed and more comfortable in her body than she could ever remember. Yet she couldn't give up one fear-driven habit: weighing herself several times each week. Her fear was that if she didn't weigh herself regularly, the old weight would creep right back on. She felt as though her positive changes would be suddenly wiped out if she ate one big meal or a slice of cake. Although she was saying all the right words, and taking many positive actions, the fear-based action was telling her unconscious mind: "I don't believe it. This success is only temporary, and it won't last."

Every time Gilda stepped on the scale, she got stressed and discouraged, which resulted in her skipping her new positive habits. Since she saw how counterproductive this compulsive weighing was to her goals, she finally decided to stop weighing herself. It was hard at first, but she found that she was more at peace with her body. Though she didn't know her weight, she did know that her clothing size remained constant and that she felt comfortable in her own skin. Food and eating became less stressful because she wasn't worrying constantly about how each morsel of food would impact the number on the scale. She found that her eating began to regulate itself. Some days she ate more than others, some days she ate less than others, but overall, she ate an appropriate amount for the size and shape of her body.

Here are some other examples of how your actions might be sending mixed messages to your mind/body system:

#1: Desire *Doesn't Match* Action	
Desire	**Action**
Stress-Free Slimness	Hurrying, rushing, checking.
Self-love, Self-acceptance	Ignoring self-care, putting off your needs, canceling appointments for self-care but not for others.
Make peace with food	Overeat/under eat. Makes food a focal point in life. You're always at war.

#2: Desire *Matches* Action	
Desire	**Action**
Stress-Free Slimness	Eat slow, enjoy food, savor the flavor. Follow the Stress-Free Slimming Strategies.
Self-love, Self-acceptance	Forgive self for all "imperfections," accept ALL parts of you, take good care of your body, mind and spirit.
Make peace with food	Eating when hungry. Listening to your body's needs.

When the desire and action don't match, you cancel out the full potential of your efforts because one cancels out the other just like a negative integer cancels out a positive integer in algebra.

Food Only Has the Power You Give It

Restrictive dieting and deprivation creates a climate of personal powerlessness. When you turn your most basic choices of what you eat and how you treat yourself over to a "diet expert," you turn your own power over and in essence say, "I don't know how to make choices, so I need someone else to make them for me." One of the first steps in reclaiming your power over food is to stop thinking of foods in terms of "good or bad," and "can have or can't have." Instead, begin thinking in terms of choice. You can choose not to eat certain foods, but it is *always your choice.* You are the one who decides to eat or not eat. You are the one who decides to buy or not buy. Food doesn't do anything but sit there until you decide to take action.

A second step in reclaiming your power over food is to begin telling yourself, "I am in control of my choices. I have a choice regarding what I eat and what I don't eat. I have power over food." In order to stop the struggle with food and your weight, you will need to acknowledge that *you are not powerless over food.* As much as you might truly feel as if you're powerless, the truth is, *you give food all the power it has.* Many times, the food we told ourselves was "bad," or a "no-no," or "off limits," is the food that has the most power over us.

When most people go on a diet, they swear off all their favorites. By definition they are only eating foods that would be their second, third or fourth choice. Well, it's no wonder that the food you'll never have again has suddenly become very desirable. We often want exactly what we can't have. Think about it, what logical person would willingly give up their favorite anything forever?

Are you willing to give up your favorite bicycle, favorite sweater, favorite collectable or hobby forever? I sure hope not. That's what makes you who you are. That's what adds enjoyment to your life. You should never surrender it forever. But you may have to put it in check. As a child, perhaps you took risks like skating without a helmet or jumping out of a tree, but you simply can't do things like that when you're an adult and expect to be healthy and injury-free. So, think in terms of how you can embrace and indulge your food favorites in moderation. Consider how you can reacquaint yourself with other passions in life so that food is no longer your only reward.

Some of us feel as though food has us in its grip and won't let go. The truth is, food has no power whatsoever except that which we assign to it. Food cannot make you buy it. Food does not prepare itself. Food doesn't fly off the table and into your mouth. The only way food can affect you is if you allow it to. For example, perhaps pasta has you in its grip because it's "bad" and you really "shouldn't" eat it. This belief automatically assigns a special power to pasta, which in turn only sets up a deprivation response, wherein the very thing you try to avoid is the thing you crave the most. If you allowed yourself to eat and enjoy all foods, eventually you would neutralize the power you previously assigned to "bad" foods. If you give yourself the power to choose, you might find that your cravings disappear. Some find that they still eat the previously "bad" food, but in much smaller quantities and with less frequency because when you know you can have any food anytime you want, it loses power and you don't feel the need to "eat it while you can."

Food is simply a mixture of various ingredients or nutrients in numerous forms. Flour has no power, nuts have no power, and chocolate has no power. These are inanimate, unconscious properties that mean nothing until we assign them meaning. Food only feels powerful because of our beliefs about it, and because of our past associations with it bringing us comfort, pleasure, guilt, and so on. For instance, when Sara talked in her Donate Your Weight support group about her addiction to a hard-to-find nut spread she ate daily as a child, the other members of the group look puzzled because they didn't even know what she was talking about. It wasn't that the nut spread was addictive itself, but rather that Sara felt addicted to how eating it made her feel safe. Over time, she was able to identify other things that brought her a sense of safety, and the nut spread just went back to being a food she enjoyed eating every once in a while, instead of an all-powerful force in her life.

If you've ever traveled to another country or engaged in a multi-cultural party, you'll see that different people like different foods and you'll understand that our likes, dislikes and cravings are tied to our experiences, not the food itself. Think about your binge foods or your food challenges. How do those foods make you feel? Why do you think they *seem* so powerful? Is this food associated with a special or significant time in life? Are you seeking comfort, safety, love, security? How can you give that to yourself? Really give yourself what you want instead of using food as a substitute. What is it you're trying to feel from eating that food, and how might you otherwise be able to feel it?

As overpowered as you might feel in this moment by any particular food item, the truth is that you have all the power in the relationship. If the food itself had actual powers, then so many people would be compelled to binge on it that there would probably be a shortage at the store. If Twinkies were addictive, you might occasionally hear of a food-related shooting where a man in Los Angeles tried to hoard twenty cases of Twinkies and a local gang tried to steal the supply.

Whatever your binge food is, no matter how delicious or spectacular or emotion-provoking it is to you, there are many people in this world who don't like it at all. There are even more people who are completely uninterested or unaware the food even exists. In fact, some have never eaten it in their entire life, nor do they have the desire to. So why does that food have no power over them, when it feels like it's ruling your life? It's because your story about the food gives it the power. Go back in history, try to remember a time when you first saw or ate this food. No doubt, it was a tie-in to an event, or series of events, in the past. But the past is over, and you can choose to change your food associations and take back your power. You can even choose to allow yourself certain off limit foods every once in a while when the craving is intense. And, you can choose to eat this food with Stress-Free Slimming Strategy #1 in mind: *Bite, Chew, Swallow, Wait.* Sit down and eat your "no-no" food slowly and consciously. Savor the flavor. Be aware of the experience. This way you are truly able to get the craving over with and get on with life.

If You Can Envision it, You Can Achieve it

The body you have today has a lot to do with the thoughts and expectations you've had over the past years of your life. If you "see" yourself as fat and frumpy, you're more likely to engage in behaviors and attitudes that create that reality. Alternatively, if you envision yourself slender and strong, you're more likely to implement positive food choices and embrace a new exercise plan that will create a strong and slender body. If you think of yourself as thin and light, you'll gravitate to choices that make that a reality for you. In this section, you'll learn multiple techniques for creating a positive self-fulfilling prophecy for your health and your life, including self-affirmative advertisements (in the form of beneficial billboards and self-fulfilling scrapbooks), visualizations, and creating history journals. When you consistently employ these techniques, you improve your chances of long-lasting, permanent weight release and good health.

Self-Affirmative Advertisements

Display advertising is extremely successful in affecting our buying behavior. Advertisers spend billions of dollars each year strategically placing billboards, bus signs, magazine and Internet ads in the right places so that we'll want to purchase their products. These images are chosen carefully to evoke emotion and desire. For many of us, the emotion evoked by women's advertising is one of, "I'm not good enough." According to a research article published in the *International Journal of Eating Disorders from the Department of Psychology*, at Kenyon College in Gambier, Ohio (Lisa M. Groesz, Michael P. Levine & Sarah K. Murnen, 1999), "Body image was significantly more negative after viewing thin media images than after viewing images of either average size models, plus size models, or inanimate objects. This effect was stronger for between-subjects designs, participants less than 19 years of age, and for participants who are vulnerable to activation of a thinness schema." The impact of media images is powerfully affecting people young and old. It doesn't seem to matter to the subconscious mind that today's media images are heavily airbrushed and out of the realm of attainable reality, or that many of the models later admit they had painful eating disorders or drug addictions, or even if those models are healthy. Our subconscious mind seems to ignore the fact that it takes hours of make-up, lighting, and Photo-Shopping to get them to look the way they do in those ads. We unconsciously internalize the idea that if only we could "get it together," (perhaps by buying a certain product), we, too, could be "perfect." We feel not good enough and we see the image before us as proof of that. Therein ensues a series of negative thoughts like, "Maybe if I reduced my fine lines/had shinier lips/lost 50 pounds/got liposuction/had thicker eyelashes/etc. etc., blah, blah, blah, then I'd feel good about myself and have everything I want in life."

These kinds of media images are powerful, but guess what? Your own thoughts are even more powerful! You can steal the media's mass-market approaches and use them to your benefit, and it will only cost you a few dollars and a few hours of your time. You can make your own advertisements and become conscious in deciding what you want to "buy." You can choose to focus on the positive outcome you crave, and pair that with the power of repetition, making sure that you see the positive images and words that support you far more than you see the ones that make you think that you need to buy something to be okay.

I recommend creating two types of self-affirmative advertisements: Beneficial Billboards and Self-Fulfilling Scrapbooks.

Beneficial Billboards

Your Beneficial Billboard can work like a multimillion-dollar ad campaign, yet the whole project can be very inexpensive, especially when you consider the return on investment. This poster-sized collage will contain words, phrases, and pictures that remind you of your goals and dreams. It's a hands-on creative project that can awaken your subconscious mind to new, positive possibilities.

To begin, you'll need a poster board, glue, a stack of magazines, some colored markers, and, if available, color copies of you at a time when you felt good in your body. Use colorful poster board that evokes a feeling of lightness and positivity.

Start by setting aside some time to sort through the magazines and cut out the words and pictures that represent positive, realistic representations of your goals. Think of how you will feel, or how you want to feel, when you release your excess weight. Choose pictures and words that symbolize exactly what you hope to attain by losing weight. Avoid pictures that you might use to beat yourself up or compare yourself unfavorably to some unrealistic expectation. Keep all the focus on what you do want, not what you don't want. For example, if part of your motivation for releasing weight is to avoid diseases such as cancer, don't put the actual word "cancer" on your collage. You don't want cancer, you want health!

You can be creative or abstract with your images and choose pictures that symbolize your goals. For example, a cat can be symbolic of autonomy, confidence, and self-esteem. A bald eagle can be symbolic of power, vision, and rare beauty.

Space your pictures enough so it's easy to focus on each one individually. Use your computer to type out your favorite words using a large font size, and search for images that inspire you and print them out. If you have a color printer, even better! Go wild and have fun and as you customize your billboard, this positive action will make changes on a deep, cellular and subconscious level. If that sounds too good to be true remember, this kind of subconscious or subliminal change has been impacting you your entire life, every time you see an advertiser's billboard. Now it's your time to decide to harness this influential power and use it in a way that works for you. Make sure your Beneficial Billboard will be enjoyable and inspiring to look at.

Once your Beneficial Billboard is complete and you feel really good about it, put it someplace where you'll be able to see it on a regular basis. Think "high traffic." Advertisers don't waste their time and money placing ads where people won't see them multiple times, because they know that advertising is not nearly as effective the first time we see it as it is the fifth, tenth, or twentieth time. Repetition is an extremely important part of this process, so place your Beneficial Billboard in a location where you'll see it daily, and allow the pictures to come to life for you. Imagine yourself doing, being and having all the elements of your Beneficial Billboard. As you imagine this vividly, your mind will open the way for these dreams to become your reality.

In the beginning, you may doubt that this strategy is going to work, but don't give up. Keep looking at your Beneficial Billboard every day until it becomes comfortable for you to think of yourself as a person who is worthy and capable of the goals you've outlined. With repeated exposure to this self-fulfilling advertisement, your new goals will begin to feel more feasible and attainable. You'll begin to feel comfortable with these new ideas, and soon you'll start feeling driven to accomplish them. You will start taking the action steps necessary to make your pictured desires a physical reality. This is the power of repetition working in your favor.

Self-Fulfilling Scrapbooks

Self-Fulfilling Scrapbooks are based on the same concept as Beneficial Billboards. The difference is that rather than putting your goals on a poster board, you put them in a book. This way, you can browse the pages of your Self-Fulfilling Scrapbook in the same way you might browse the pages of a magazine. Use an attractive notebook, scrapbook, or photo album with removable pages so you can move pictures around and add new items easily. As you work with this book, you'll undoubtedly want to add and delete pictures. Your goals will start coming true and you won't need to focus on them as intently. You also might decide to change your goals, realizing your original goal wasn't quite right for you.

Take time to find images for your Scrapbook that really get you motivated and make you feel excited and anticipatory. Avoid using small, drab, colorless, or worn-out pictures. Put in pictures of people being active, eating healthily, and enjoying the activities you want to enjoy. Draw or paint images and words that are focused on everything you want to come true in your life.

Once you've designed a Self-Fulfilling Scrapbook, make a commitment to look through it daily at a relaxed pace. It won't do you any good if it remains closed and sitting on a desk somewhere. You must look at it daily and look at it with hope, positive expectation, and enthusiasm.

As you look at your Self-Fulfilling Scrapbook and/or Beneficial Billboard each day, you'll probably start to experience small changes in your thinking and your behavior. As time passes, you'll notice yourself moving closer and closer to your goals without much stress or strain. You have absolutely nothing to lose from this practice and quite a bit to gain, so give it a try. If you believe that it's possible for you to have all of these things in your life, you will slowly start to take the actions needed for you to have them.

You may want to look through the Self-Fulfilling Scrapbook while pretending that today is actually the future. Pretend that as you browse the pages, you are actually looking back on all of the things you've done in life. Pretend you're thinking about old times, just like you probably do now with old photos of your family and friends. Acting as if the goals depicted in your Scrapbook have already come true can focus your unconscious mind on how to make them happen. Choose a supportive friend who you trust and share your Scrapbook with him or her. Pretend you're going over memories and say things like, "This is me in my bathing suit in the Bahamas."

Children are good at daydreaming and making up fun scenarios. As adults we can become too logical for our own good, getting stuck in the roles and rigid rules we've set for ourselves and forgetting to have fun. Try not to take yourself too seriously. You don't have to know all the details of how you'll accomplish your goals. If you put the intention out there and focus on it daily, ideas and inspirations will come to you in unexpected ways. Someday that Self-Fulfilling Scrapbook will be a true record of the things you've done in your life.

Relaxation and Visualization Techniques

In addition to having external visual reminders of our desires and goals, it's also incredibly powerful to use visualization techniques to picture in our mind's eye what we want to accomplish. These techniques require only an open mind and imagination, and the more often you do them, the quicker and more lasting your success will be.

For some people, visualization feels challenging at first, but everyone will sharpen this skill with practice. Try practicing this technique at least six times before you decide whether or not it will work for you. Spread your six attempts over a two-week period. If you give this technique a genuine shot, and it still doesn't suit your personality, taste, and style, you can just set this technique aside. Perhaps you might decide to revisit it at a later time.

The key to using the imagination is relaxation. The more you can relax, the more effective the upcoming visualization techniques will be for you. Since deep relaxation is a skill that improves with practice, simply recognize that it might take some time before you can really hone this skill and harness its full power. Have no fear, if you're willing, patient and persistent your relaxation skills will improve.

Getting Relaxed

Begin by reflecting on what relaxation techniques are already working for you or have worked for you in the past. Sit quietly, reflect, and write "things that help me feel relaxed" on the top of a blank sheet of paper. Then, continue to sit quietly and reflect. No pressure. Give yourself time. Each time you think of something, write it down. The reward ideas at the end of Chapter 4 might help you get a jumpstart. Give yourself a week to focus on relaxation and what helps you to relax. Keep the list handy so you can add to it anytime you like.

Once you've identified the things that help you relax, your next order of business is to integrate those relaxing activities into your daily life. Practice your ability to relax. Begin creating an environment that reminds you to relax. For example, if the sound of running water helps you relax, get a fountain or an environmental sounds CD. If scents help you relax, keep lotions, candles, fresh flowers, incense, or other scented items readily available and use them often. If beautiful images are relaxing, try to place your favorite pieces in a place where you will see them often. If watching fire helps you relax, light candles or sit near a fireplace. If being with animals or pets calms you down, spend time with them and put pictures or trinkets in your environment that remind you of them. If vacation is relaxing, be sure to put photos or reminders of your favorite places within your line of sight. If spending time outdoors is relaxing, try to schedule activities that take place outdoors.

Practice with purposeful relaxation daily. Spend ten to fifteen minutes each morning focusing on relaxation. Recall relaxing times and make it your intention to recreate those feelings. Imagine the feeling of relaxation vividly. Create a relaxing environment and notice how your body responds. With practice, you will get better and better and be able to relax quicker and more easily. Don't worry or fret about wasting time (self-care is *never* a waste of time!), and tell yourself, "I'm getting better and better at relaxation each and every day."

If it seems hard to relax at first, don't give up. Even if it seems that nine of the ten minutes you set aside for relaxation were really a "waste of time," don't worry. It will absolutely, positively be worth your time to hang in there. Turn your one minute of success into two minutes, and then into five, until you find that all ten minutes feel pretty relaxing and refreshing.

Each day you practice relaxing you'll get stronger, and you will soon begin reaping the benefits of being in greater control of your life. You will cease to be a "responder" who reacts to cues from others, and you will begin to be a creator who decides what you do and don't want in your life.

Learning to Visualize

Once you improve your relaxation skills, you can purposely begin to use your periods of relaxation to focus on and create the future goals you desire. I will provide you with a few sample visualizations to get started. I recommend that you spend purposeful, dedicated time rehearsing these visualizations each day, and also allow yourself to recall the images at random throughout the day during "down time," such as when you're using the restroom, cooking, cleaning, applying make-up, etc.

When you practice visualization, keep in mind that it's fine to either sense the images or actually "see" them as pictures in your mind. The impact of either is as powerful, or more powerful, than anything you might say to yourself. Going back to the marketing analogy, you'll notice that advertisers use as few words as possible to convey their message. Instead, they rely heavily on images that will evoke emotion, spark an association, or elicit desire and yearning. Images are powerful. They transcend culture, language, class, and creeds. Many of us have been touched on a deep level by photos and paintings of people and places we know nothing about. Images are a universal language, and your ability to understand and utilize images can be an important part of your weight release program. Below are some sample visualizations to help get you started.

Sample Visualization #1: Speedy Metabolism and Efficient Digestion

Have you ever said, "All I have to do is look at food and I gain weight?" If you have, it's likely that your body took that as a command, and that's not the kind of mind-body understanding you want to create for yourself. Instead, it's time to begin purposely deciding which thoughts you'll use to feed your mind.

Imagine that your body is a high-functioning processing plant with a series of smooth-running departments. As soon as food is delivered to your system, a team of workers analyze the delivery and begin to categorize the contents. All vitamins and minerals are delivered to the locations where they're needed most. The energy that is needed in that moment from the food is delivered to your mind and your limbs and all excess calories are immediately delivered to the digestive system where they are broken down into small pieces and whisked down the chute to your large intestines. From there, these excess calories twist and turn down the roller coaster of your winding small intestine and are delivered to the waste department.

Did you see the *I Love Lucy* episode where Lucy and Ethyl are working at the chocolate factory? Remember how the conveyor belt begins to speed up and Lucy can't keep up with her part of the assembly line. She begins to tuck candies in her dress and things get crazy. If you overload your body with excess calories, it will clog up and slow the entire system down. On the flipside, if the food is coming in at a steady rate and the processing department is able to keep up with incoming food, everything runs smoothly. If you've overloaded the system for many years, you have backlog, and the processing team will have no other choice but to store the backlog of excess calories as fat until the intake slows down enough for them to get back to processing the excess. Now imagine that you've hired an additional team to help out: the clean-up crew. Their job is to go get the stored fat, break it up, and send it into the digestive system for processing.

For ease and speed, the crew will also burn some of the fat storage, just like farmers sometimes burn their crops to clear the land. Imagine the bulky fat beginning to melt and disintegrate, as the flame gets hot. The remnants are then sent down the chute for further processing.

Continue this visualization daily and when you use the restroom, gleefully imagine the fat being whisked away to its new destination. As this processing plant becomes a daily part of your awareness, you can start to help it be even more efficient by doing the following:

1. Cut down on the amount you put into the system so you can give it a better chance to catch up with the backlog.
2. Chew slowly so that food can digest more efficiently.
3. Give the system some rest (time off) so it can revitalize and come back to work more efficiently. Research indicates that lack of sleep can be a factor in weight problems and overeating. (*USA Today*, 2004)
4. Help the system speed up by exercising and moving about. This helps energize your metabolism so food is processed quickly.
5. Help whisk the fat through your system more quickly by continually flushing it out with water.

You are the CEO of your processing plant. It is your job to analyze the process and continually look for ways to streamline the operation and improve the overall functioning. Keep a close eye on things and adjust as necessary. Find what works best and keep doing it, and you can't help but succeed. The Donate

Your Weight CD: *Rev Up Your Metabolism* will also aid you in visualizing a rapid metabolism and can help you feel more motivated to take positive actions.

Sample Visualization #2: Cleaning out Your Mental/Emotional Garage

Many of us hold on to excess weight for reasons that have little or no correlation to our current eating or exercise habits. For some, the extra weight represents heavy emotions that are "stuck" in our bodies like hair might get stuck in a drain. I believe that removing these emotional blocks can facilitate the body in functioning more efficiently. The following visualization will help you clean out your mental and emotional blocks, leaving you with a clear pathway to thoughts and behaviors that will result in the creation of the body you desire.

Imagine in your mind's eye that your body is a storage space that resembles a garage. Imagine that all of your past wounds, unresolved pains, and repressed emotions have taken the form of boxes. These boxes are filled up and piled high, and you haven't looked in many of them for years. As you relax deeply, allow your imagination to create a scene that matches your personal situation. If there's just one big issue you feel like you haven't resolved, perhaps your garage only has one box in it. If you know that are myriad issues and pains hanging around, your garage may be packed full. It's possible that some of the items in the boxes are very valuable, important, and worth saving, but it's likely that some of the boxes are filled with unnecessary junk, perhaps that you haven't used in years and will never again be needed or useful.

It's time to free yourself from the weight of this clutter. Open a box and take a good look at the contents inside. If this feels overwhelming, see if a friend or therapist will keep you company while you do this visualization. And don't feel like you have to go through all the boxes in one sitting. You can start with a small one labeled, "Minor hurts," or, "Things I can handle," or you perhaps your boxes will be labeled by the years of your life or by the relationship they connect to (yourself, your parents, friends, coworkers, the mean guy at the auto repair shop, etc.).

Promise yourself that you'll only look inside boxes when you feel ready and safe to do so. Remind yourself that cleaning out these boxes will make room for all the things you want in your life that you don't presently have "space" for. You can repeat this visualization regularly, until you are able to have boxes only for things you want to keep in your life, leaving you with tons of space for healthy habits, plenty of self-care, and positive and loving relationships.

Before you open each box, say to yourself. "I am now releasing, eliminating, and letting go of all old items that no longer suit me. As I release and let go, I become lighter and freer." Then open the lid of the box and survey the contents.

Pull out each item one by one, really looking at each one closely and asking yourself:

- Does this serve me well?
- Does this make me happy?
- Does this make me a better person?
- Does this enhance my life?
- Do I want this?

If you can easily answer "yes" to each of these questions, you can put this item in a beautiful case labeled "Things Worth Keeping." But if your answer is "no," allow yourself to take this item outside the garage and put it in a dumpster. Tell yourself, "I am now willing to release this. I am ready to let go and to choose only what's in my best interests." Sometimes when letting items go, you may have flashes of inspirations, ideas, or images. Write these down after your visualization session.

If there are certain items you feel ambivalent about, put them into a box marked "Undecided." It may be that you wait until the end to go through this box again, perhaps with the help of someone you trust. Tell yourself, "I am open to help from others, and I am ready to let go."

At the end of each visualization session, imagine friendly garbage collectors coming and emptying out your dumpster, carrying away your unwanted items, and leaving you with an empty dumpster for the next time you do this visualization. Say to yourself, "What I am setting into motion in my mind's eye will slowly start to help me create the changes I want in my life. I will get what I need when I need it, and I am committed to clearing out my garage until all I'm left with is what truly serves me, enhances my life's happiness, allows me to be my best self."

Sample Visualization #3: See Yourself Successfully Using the Seven Stress-Free Slimming Strategies

Another effective and powerful way to use visualization is to vividly imagine yourself doing things in a new way. If you can see and believe your goals and dreams, you can achieve them. This is true of everything in life, including breaking lifelong habits and transforming your body and/or body image. The more time you spend vividly imagining yourself doing things a new way, the easier it will be to eventually make the changes you desire. In fact, with repeated and purposeful use of visualizations, you are likely to notice small, gradual, and easy changes in your behavior, almost as if they're happening automatically.

After you have rehearsed something many times in your mind, you will be prepared for the actual situation when it arises, just like you'll find yourself standing in a doorway for an earthquake or you would automatically get under your desk in the case of a fire drill. When you imagine and practice success, you'll find yourself capable of doing the very things you imagined yourself doing. Following is a visualization that can help you succeed in integrating the Seven Stress-Free Slimming Strategies into your daily life.

Imagine that as soon as you wake up in the morning, you start drinking water. You like to be refreshed and revitalized. You find it easy to drink 48 ounces of water every day. After you drink some water, you get ready for your morning exercise. You love the energy and strength you get from exercise. You picture yourself doing your favorite exercise, appreciating yourself and your body for being active. Before you know it, you've completed your twenty minutes of exercise and it's time to take a shower. As you shower, you say your positive affirmations to yourself. You sing your affirmations. You see yourself succeeding at your goals. You make a commitment to do something fun and frivolous for yourself today. Whether it's stopping to smell a rose, going window shopping, taking a bath, or getting a pedicure, you know you will take time for yourself and that as a result, you will feel cared for and more fulfilled.

You dry off and go to the kitchen to prepare yourself a healthy breakfast. You enjoy the process of making yourself a healthy meal, because you know that doing so is a great way to take care of yourself and that it will pay off in all areas of your life. You fix your plate and sit down to eat it. You first look at your food, determining if it looks and smells appealing. Pretend that you are a professional tester, and that only the freshest, healthiest meal will do. Observe your breakfast, and determine if it's worthy of putting in your mouth and your stomach. Imagine that this food passes your most rigorous tests for healthiness and good taste and smell.

Now bring the first bite to your mouth, noticing the aroma. As you open your mouth, you take a small and delicate bite. Notice the reaction from your taste buds. Savor the range of flavors. Is it sweet, salty, spicy, or tangy? Notice the nuances of the food item as you begin to chew. Chew slowly and methodically. Chew as if you have nothing better to do. Chew as if you have all the time in the world. Feel the strength and sexiness of your body as you take your time nourishing it. Continue to chew the food until it dissolves in your mouth. Swallow thoroughly and pause before you take your second bite. You are in no hurry. You've set aside plenty of time to nourish your body because you know it's important to your overall health and well-being. Being healthy and well-nourished helps you to accomplish and achieve everything that's important to you. You enjoy lingering over your meal and taking your time.

As you continue eating, eventually you notice that you have had enough food. You are satisfied. You stop prior to becoming "full," because you don't desire or deserve to ever feel "stuffed." There is still food on your plate, but since you are satisfied, you push the plate away with food still on it and refuse to take even one bite past your comfort zone. After all, this is your body, you want what's best for it. You do something wonderful just for you. It could be as small as clipping a fresh flower for your desk or taking a day off to go to the spa. Spend time closing your eyes and getting into a relaxed, hypnotic state. Allow this visualization to come in full color as if you're watching High Definition Television. Allow yourself to feel what it's like to live your life in a new and healthy way every day. For added support in visualizing yourself successfully implementing the Slimming Strategies, you can also purchase the Stress-Free Slimming CD from Donate Your Weight.

Sample Visualization #4: See Yourself Where You Want to Be

Your mind and body respond to the images you focus on. Imagine you have reached your weight-release goal. Imagine yourself stepping on the scale and seeing your goal number. See yourself trying on a smaller size of clothing and imagine that it fits perfectly. Notice how you carry yourself. Notice your posture. How do you feel emotionally? How do you feel physically? How do your arms feel? How do you feel in your clothes? What changes do you notice in your hips, stomach, back, and buttocks? Notice everything in vivid detail. Get as specific as you can. Really get into this feeling of being slimmer and trimmer. Hold this feeling and image of yourself at your ideal weight for five to ten minutes, and just feel the pleasure of having taken such good care of yourself that you are fit, healthy and energetic. Go on with your day, holding this feeling and image in the back of your mind as the person you are becoming. "Act the part" of someone you admire. Pretend you are living the life you always wanted to live. What does your body feel like? Feel your shoulders upright, your posture straight, your head held high.

If you struggle with this visualization, perhaps it's because you have never actually felt like you were at an ideal or comfortable weight, or maybe you've never felt confidence about your body. Try this variation: Think of a slender and strong person you admire who is close to your age and has a similar body style to yours in terms of proportions. Imagine you are in that body, walking around tall and proud and feeling the same feelings you would have if that were currently your body.

Now imagine all the ways people respond to this new you. When someone asks, "Have you lost weight?" answer "Yes, I have released weight. Thanks for noticing." (By the way, this is *always* the way to respond when someone asks this question.) Notice that you say "I *have released* weight," not, "I *am losing* weight," (which isn't as specific and immediate as the first statement) or "No, I haven't lost weight," (which is like an anti-affirmation to your mind). Help your body achieve success more quickly and easily by affirming and supporting the results you desire.

Cheer yourself on for having this fabulously comfortable, sexy, and healthy body. Tell yourself, "I believe in myself and I embrace my strengths." As you come out of this visualization, hold on to the feeling and image of having this great body and confident attitude. Walk and talk like this is the body you already have, and continue to do this visualization/affirmation/action combination daily. By doing so, you will absolutely look and feel better within thirty to sixty days.

Creating History Journals

Writing a Creating History Journal can help you create personalized visualizations and set them into motion by making a tangible representation of "the truth told in advance." This journal will work somewhat like affirmations, except it will be a little more free-flowing and creative. Plus, it will evoke positive feelings of joy that will propel you to your goals more quickly than just saying words. It'll also be more descriptive, much in the same style as a journal or diary, except that it will actually be about your life a year in the future.

Get yourself an attractive, stately and visually pleasing notebook or diary and enter in today's day and month with next year's year. Then begin writing what your day and your life looks like. Write in the same style as you would in a regular journal, describing things as if they are happening now (such as, "I feel so great about my body,") or as they happened earlier in the day (such as, "I had a great time exercising today"). In this entry, you may want to imagine yourself reaching a weight release goal. Choose a reasonable goal weight or size for a year from now. According to the Partnership for Healthy Weight Maintenance, a multidisciplinary team of professional and governmental agencies[1], "For safe and healthy weight loss, try not to exceed a rate of two pounds per week." So if you want to lose 50 pounds, give yourself at least 6 months to a year. On the date of your first entry, you may want to write about how you feel now that you've reached your goal. Here is an example:

---

1   http://www.consumer.gov/weightloss/setgoals.htm

June 23

    I am so proud and satisfied. I stepped on the scale today and I am exactly at my goal weight. It feels fantastic. All of the clothes that I used to wear are all too big for me now—even my rings and my watch are too big! I really feel so much better in my body. I think I will go shopping today and buy myself some new clothes. People are really beginning to notice the changes. Just today two people said something about how great I look. I feel great, too. I don't ever want to gain that weight back again. This is a very comfortable system for me and I will maintain it for the rest of my life. I love getting regular exercise, eating and drinking healthily and thoughtfully, and no longer putting myself on yo-yo diets that never worked for me and just made me feel miserable. What a relief to be free of that awful cycle!

You can also use the Creating History Journal to imagine reaching milestones in your body image and self-esteem. Here is an example:

July 17

    I feel so much better about myself now. I remember how I used to be so hard on myself that I couldn't even think of one thing I liked about myself. Today, I was able to come up with a list of ten good things about myself and I really did believe each of them on a deep level. I have compassion for my vulnerabilities and struggles, and I can actually accept myself, flaws and all. Yea for me!!!

You can also use the journal to imagine yourself doing things a new way. For example:

August 24

    Today I looked at a plate of pizza and I must say, I wasn't even tempted to eat it. It actually looked greasy to me and I knew that if I ate it, I would probably feel sick to my stomach. It wasn't even a battle at all. I just decided not to eat it and I felt so powerful. I really do have power over food and it feels great.

As you can see, a Creating History Journal helps you focus on positive outcomes rather than worrying and focusing on worst-case scenarios. Some of us have actually kept journals and when we read them over, we find that they're actually just a litany of all that's wrong with us and our lives. While it can be useful to express your painful feelings through journaling, the purpose of a Creating History Journal is to intentionally keep your focus on what you want and imagine it all coming true. While writing, be careful not to get stuck on particular details of how things must go. Simply imagine positive outcomes and positive feelings. Write about your ideal day in as much vivid detail as possible. Include feelings, sights, sounds, smells, and anything that will make that journal entry come alive for you.

Sitting down and writing this journal will actually serve as a sort of salve, soothing past times of harshness and negativity with yourself and drawing out more and more positive thoughts and feelings. This process will allow you to change your perspective and begin creating the life you want. It's a purposeful exercise that helps you draw to yourself what you want, because as the saying goes, "You are what you think about all day long." Use the Creating History Journal to help you become the person you want to be.

PART II

CREATING AN
ACTION PLAN
FOR A THINNER,
HEALTHIER YOU

CHAPTER 4

THE SEVEN STRESS-FREE SLIMMING STRATEGIES

The Seven Stress-Free Slimming Strategies can help you become naturally slimmer and stop the struggle with weight and eating. Be forewarned: they are incredibly simple and even enjoyable. If you're still stuck in a diet mentality or a "no pain, no gain" mindset, you may jump to conclusions or judge these steps as "too simple." You might also find yourself saying, "I already tried that" or sarcastically rolling your eyes and muttering under your breath, "If only it was that easy." Well, guess what, it is this easy.

If you're coming from a history of numerous diets and numerous failures, you are used to suffering. You may only feel like its "working" if you are hungry, weak, deprived, or losing weight rapidly. But let's face it, that type of weight release has always been temporary and it always will be. Using that model, you may have even gained back more weight than you lost, which means that the diet that supposedly "worked" actually set you back instead of helping you get healthier. The dieting cycle may have left you feeling like a terrible failure who will never have the healthy, energetic body you want.

If this is the case, take heart. Now that you know better, you can do better. You don't have to keep making the same mistakes over and over. As you read the following steps and begin incorporating them into your life, dare to keep an open mind. Refuse to sabotage your success by saying, "It will never work." Instead, tell yourself, "It will work because I will do what it takes to make it work!" Aren't you sick of being miserable? Aren't you sick of deprivation? Wouldn't you love to have a life that's free from self-hatred and criticism, free from food and weight obsession?

These seven simple strategies will get you to the weight you desire if you commit to them and refuse to give up. Below is the rhyming version of the strategies. Read them daily to help you memorize the steps easily and create a positive, playful association with your life-long journey to weight maintenance.

1.   Bite, Chew, Swallow, Wait;
2.   Leave Some Food on Your Plate;
3.   Drink Your Water 6x8;
4.   Exercise for 20, 3 to 5 days;
5.   Feed Your Mind, Change What You Say;
6.   Do Self-Hypnosis Every Day; and
7.   Pamper Yourself, Don't Delay.

These steps are outlined in detail in Appendix 3 for your convenience or you can download a full-color list of these strategies to put on your refrigerator or near your desk at http://www.donateyourweight.com/images/7strat.pdf.

Notice that the Seven Stress-Free Slimming Strategies is a list of things you can do, not a list of things you *can't* or *mustn't* do. Already, this approach is more positive than dieting. Diets ultimately end up being about deprivation. When you talk to someone on a diet, they say "I can't have that," "That food is bad," or, "I have to eat this boring rabbit food." The feelings related to being on a diet are most often misery, depression, sadness, self-pity, and boredom. It's more common to hear someone complain about a diet than to be excited about it. If you go to lunch with someone on a diet, they usually order a salad as they admire the food on other people's plates. They sigh and slump their shoulders as they shove one more forkful of greens into their mouth. They aren't feeling free or having fun, acting instead like they're in prison. How long do you think any logical human being is going to be able to sustain such a tortuous program? And more importantly, why would they want to? Failing to keep to a miserable, depriving diet isn't due to a lack of willpower, it's due to a natural and sane desire not to feel miserable all day, every day, for the rest of your life.

Most dieters "cheat" or go off their diet within a short period of time. Many nutritional counselors, educators and even registered dieticians have stopped putting their clients on diets and started teaching them to have a new relationship with food. Evelyn Tribole and Elyse Resch are both registered dieticians with successful practices. In their book, *Intuitive Eating–A Revolutionary Program that Works* (1995) they share the numerous stories and anecdotes about their clients that caused them to change their minds about dieting. They decided to give up on prescribing diets to their clients after seeing the continual failures, feelings of defeat, obsessive behavior, unhappiness and unhealthy behavior that resulted from dieting. They now adopt a 100% diet-free model in their practices with much success.

The American Obesity Association[2] a subsidiary of the Federal Trade Commission in Washington D.C., states: "The truth is that if there really is a miracle cure, 64.5 percent of adult Americans would not be overweight." The following thought-provoking statistics are available at their website:

- "Consumers spend about $30 billion per year trying to lose weight or prevent weight gain. This figure includes spending on diet sodas, diet foods, artificially sweetened products, appetite suppressants, diet books, videos and cassettes, medically supervised and commercial programs, and fitness clubs.
- Spending on weight loss programs is estimated at $1 to $2 billion per year.
- U.S. food manufacturers are estimated to have spent $7 billion on advertising of highly processed and packaged foods in 1997."

So can we just agree that quick-fix diets don't work? We must make sustainable lifestyle changes if we want permanent results. The Seven Stress-Free Slimming Strategies that follow can help make the process of becoming and staying slim easy and healthy. Each of the strategies has a basis in increasing health and decreasing impulsivity. Attention to these simple steps can help you break life-long habits with relative ease.

Strategy #1: Bite, Chew, Swallow, Wait

This single strategy, if followed consistently and faithfully, will almost automatically lead to eating less and losing weight. Many of us eat quickly and unconsciously, as if we're robots. We rush through meals like they're some sort of chore and barely take time to taste or enjoy the food that we're eating. This unconscious eating leads to low levels of satisfaction with the food we eat, disconnection with our body's cues, and the over-feeding our bodies—all of which result in weight gain.

Your stomach is about the size of your fist. It has the ability to stretch, but that doesn't mean that it's wise or healthy to regularly eat so much that it forces your stomach to stretch. Instead, take small bites and chew each bite at least ten times, but continue until the food dissolves in your mouth. At first, as you learn

---

2   http://obesity1.tempdomainname.com/subs/fastfacts/Obesity_Consumer_ Protect.shtml

this habit, try tapping your fingers on the table one at a time as you silently count each chew from one to ten. Chewing slowly helps break down the food, which allows your body to process and digest the food more efficiently. Waiting between bites gives your body more time to process the food, and gives your body time to send a signal to your mind when you're satisfied. If you shovel the food in your mouth nonstop, you'll find yourself stuffed before your mind ever has a chance to register that you're satisfied. This approach inevitably leads to overeating, often to the point of feeling uncomfortably full and taking even more pleasure away from the experience of eating.

So for each meal, make a conscious effort to eat slowly. The food isn't going anywhere. It will be there no matter how fast or slow you eat. If you don't finish it all now, you can put it away for later. There is no reason to shovel it all in quickly.

Strategy #2: Leave Some Food on Your Plate

In order to lose weight and keep it off, we need to learn to eat for physical hunger, not for emotional or habitual reasons. Many of us always eat until our plate is clean, even if some of it doesn't taste good to us or we start to feel full. Some of us are so entrenched in this habit that we are completely out of touch with our own bodies. If this is the case for you, consciously deciding to leave food on your plate will be an important step in becoming aware of your body. Utilizing this strategy in conjunction with strategy one ("Bite, Chew, Swallow, Wait") will automatically lead to a decrease in food intake and an increase in your food satisfaction.

The ultimate goal is to get off of automatic pilot and begin to tune in to your own body's signals for "hunger" and "satisfied." Notice I didn't say "full." If you eat to get "full", chances are you will feel "stuffed" within ten to twenty minutes. Instead, the goal is to eat until you're satisfied: that is, your hunger pangs have subsided, you feel energized and you've eaten enough food to fuel your body for three to five hours. Feeling satisfied after a meal means never feeling "stuffed." You should be able to comfortably walk about and have no need to unbutton or unzip your pants.

When you stuff yourself, you overload your body's natural digestive process. Your body has no choice but to put some of this excess food in storage to be processed later. If you continually stuff yourself, the storage gets bigger and bigger and eventually turns to fat in your body. By the same token, if you eat smaller amounts, your body can keep up with the intake and will even dip into the storage (excess fat) after it's finished processing the food you just ate.

If you're clearing your plate because there are starving children in the world, it's time for a reality check: your being overweight will do nothing to help those less fortunate. If you really want to help starving children, Donate Your Weight to them (see chapter 5) or participate in a charity campaign for hunger relief. If you've been taught to never waste any food because you "never know" if there will be enough in some unforeseeable tomorrow, realize that it's highly unlikely that you'll face starvation in your lifetime. If you've been told you are ungrateful and wasteful for not eating all your food, put tiny portions on your plate so you waste very little, and try to let that guilt-trip go. If you were told to eat all you can at buffets or restaurants to "get your money's worth," consider the long-term healthcare costs that will inevitably come with being overweight. If you had poor or frugal parents who said things like, "I paid good money for that food and you'd better eat every bite," realize that you're an adult now and you get to decide exactly what you put in your mouth.

Some of us were sternly punished for not clearing our plates, so is it any wonder that this habit is hardwired and unquestioned for many of us? But as you take a close look at the concepts in this book, you'll see that you don't "save" anything when you continually overeat. Instead, you lose. You lose power, you lose your health, and you lose your self-respect. You also "pay." You pay by being stuck with a body you don't want. You pay because you have to keep buying new clothes. You pay by feeling bad about yourself. You pay with medical problems that can create a need for medication, treatment, and sometimes even surgery. If you continue to gain weight and neglect your health, you may even pay with your own life, prematurely cutting it short due to disease.

These are all ample reasons to change your thinking about automatically cleaning your plate. Take into consideration that portions are considerably larger today than they probably were when you were a child. Not that long ago, adults and kids alike ate the Happy Meal portion of French fries at McDonald's and that was considered a serving. All bags of potato and tortilla chips for sale were the size of today's "snack size" and a 12-ounce soda was the standard size. Today, some people are carting around 44 ounce beverages. This "bigger is better" marketing mentality is pervasive in our culture, but with awareness and persistence, we can remember what the size of a healthy portion is and allow ourselves to stop eating before we go too far.

The National Heart Lung and Blood Institute website hosts a slide show and quiz to demonstrate the transformation of portion sizes over the past 20 years.[3] As an example, 20 years ago an average bagel was 3" in diameter and 140

---

3   The portion distortion slide show is available at http://hp2010.nhlbihin. net/portion/

calories. Now the average bagel is 6" in diameter and 350 calories. That's a 210 calorie difference … more than double what it used to be! No wonder we're perplexed. Maybe when you say, "I used to eat a bagel every day when I was younger and I didn't gain weight" your statement actually says more about the portion distortion than it does about your age and metabolism.

We see larger-than-life pictures of food all day long on television, on billboards, in magazines, and at restaurants. We have come to equate large portions with "a good deal," and some of us may even avoid certain restaurants because they "don't give you enough food." But the truth is, finishing everything on your plate at a restaurant can mean eating two to five servings of food. Just because a restaurant sells a plate of food as a meal, it doesn't mean that the portions and ingredients are in line with your goals of becoming a naturally slim person. Avoid the temptation to fall prey to this marketing mentality and instead honor your own body and its cues. Take extra food to-go; you can always have it later if you want. Getting off of automatic pilot when you eat will pay big dividends, not only in regard to your weight reduction goals, but also in relation to your self-esteem and self-love, because you will be listening to, and trusting yourself rather than giving your power to others.

Strategy #3: Drink Your Water 6x8

Our bodies are more than 70 percent water. Water is an important part of our survival and health. Giving your body at least 48 ounces of water each day flushes out your system, hydrates you, and helps keep your skin and hair healthy. Sometimes you may misinterpret your hunger pangs as a need for food when what your body really wants is water. Therefore, drinking water regularly might cause you to eat less.

You may think you don't need much water, or that as long as you "drink something" you're okay. But just like you can't substitute coffee for gasoline in your car, you can't substitute coffee, alcohol, or sodas for clean, clear, fresh water. You lose about ten cups of water a day through perspiration, urination, and crying. You are constantly losing water. Caffeinated beverages, such as colas or coffee, and alcoholic beverages cause dehydration and contain empty calories and unhealthy additives. If you don't replenish by drinking water, you are actually depriving your body of a necessary element for survival and health. Sure, you can exist without drinking six glasses of water a day, but there's a good chance that you will be paying a price health-wise, perhaps in small, unnoticeable ways each day. If you want an easy way to improve your health and release extra weight, drinking water is a great start.

Some of you have probably read much higher daily requirements for water intake. The truth is, according to a 2004 report from the Institute of Medicine, even 48 ounces of water a day might be too much. In a *New York Times* article, Jane Brody summarizes the report and writes, "You may not have to drink eight glasses of water a day to be well hydrated, and you can count caffeinated beverages in your total water intake, according to a new report from the Institute of Medicine, the group that sets desirable levels of nutrient intake for Americans of all ages." So, if you're one of those people who feels like a washing machine on the rinse cycle when you drink 8, eight-ounce glasses a day or, you've been trying to think of a way to cut out five of your 20 bathroom breaks, this report might be good news for you. But if you have the water habit anyway and you like the routine, keep it up.

Strategy #4: Exercise for Twenty, Three to Five Days

Oh, how often we've heard about the importance of regular exercise. It's recommended for overall health and fitness, for metabolism and blood circulation, and for a strong heart and muscles. Exercise helps us sleep better at night and wake up more refreshed, and it's even indicated as a treatment for depression and anxiety. The benefits are numerous and wide-ranging, yet some of us just can't seem to get up off the couch and do it. If you don't already exercise regularly, consider the following four points:

1. There are many enjoyable ways to get exercise.
2. Even mild to moderate exercise improves health.
3. Exercise/moving can help your metabolism run more efficiently.
4. You don't have to be a muscle-bound gym rat to get benefits from exercise.

In my years of working with people who have weight problems, I have noticed a common theme: all-or-nothing thinking. Many of us avoid exercise, or exercise sporadically, because we have an "all-or-nothing" belief system that causes us to think we must do something perfectly, or else it's not worth doing at all. We try to be perfect and when we can't be perfect, we quit. We might even make fun of exercise and pretend to be proud that we don't exercise. We might exclaim, "I hate exercise," or shudder when someone recommends it to us. Remember, life is never all or nothing—there are tons of compromises along the way, successes and setbacks, good moments and bad ones. So recognize when you're engaged in all-or-nothing thinking and shift your thoughts consciously to an alternative, more doable point of view. This is a crucial key to permanent weight-reduction success. Here are some examples of how to make the shift:

All-or-Nothing Thinking	Alternative, Doable Point of View
You have to buy all the "right" equipment and clothing first (i.e., "I need a treadmill at home," "I have to buy the right socks," "I need a new jog bra," etc.).	Exercise in whatever clothes and with whatever equipment you have available. As you progress in your routine, you can slowly get things you need to make you feel more comfortable.
You have to "look good" in your exercise outfit (i.e., "I can't exercise with this big butt! What will people think?").	Don't worry about what you look like when you exercise. The more you do it, the better you'll look. Plus, you can always exercise in private where no one will see you anyway.
You have to either join a gym or get a personal trainer (i.e., "I would exercise, but I don't have enough money to hire a personal trainer").	You can exercise anywhere, whether you stretch at your desk; do a workout video in your house; or walk or run in your backyard, your neighborhood, your local mall, etc.
You have to follow the plan perfectly or you're a lazy, hopeless, undisciplined failure.	There is no "perfect." Focus on progress, not perfection. If you don't follow it perfectly today, that's okay. Do what you can do today and try again tomorrow. This is a life-long process.
If you don't see immediate results, it's not working and you might as well "just give up," (i.e., "I've been exercising for a month now and I don't see or feel any difference. What's the point?").	*Don't give up!* Whatever you do, *don't give up!* If all you can muster is a walk around the block, *do it*! You can improve and increase later. Just do whatever you can right now and build slowly.

If you're still struggling for motivation, I'd like to challenge you to write down all your excuses for not exercising. Go ahead, put them down on paper so you can see them in black and white. After you finish writing them all down, go back and analyze them one at a time. Play devil's advocate with yourself, coming up with an argument *against* your excuse. Ask yourself, "Is this excuse really valid?" "Is there another way to look at this?" Challenge all negative, perfectionist, all-or-nothing thinking. And remember: a tiny bit of exercise is better than no exercise at all. It's perfectly acceptable to start with a daily walk around the block. Soon you will feel strong enough to increase to a two block walk. Don't expect yourself to go from sitting on the couch to running a mile a day. Be patient and realistic with yourself and oh, did I mention, *don't give up!*

If you are a self-proclaimed "couch potato", or perhaps a person who loves to exercise but still doesn't do it, here are some ideas on how get more movement/activity in your life without joining a gym or buying a workout wardrobe:

- Pull weeds,
- Scrub the floor,
- Play with the dog,
- Park farther away and walk,
- Walk when performing your errands,
- Walk in the mall,
- Put hand-weights or resistance bands near your TV and exercise during every commercial break,
- Flex your muscles while you're in line, in your car, sitting at your desk, or waiting on hold,
- Pull in your abdominal muscles throughout the day,
- Use a cordless phone or a wireless headset and pace while you talk,
- Take the stairs instead of the elevator, and
- Put a medicine ball near your computer and do arm exercises during downloads or print jobs.

I could go on and on, but I think you get the picture. Stop comparing yourself to Suzy Super Thin or Motivated Melvin and give yourself permission to start where you are and work up from there. Once you get started and comfortable with a regular routine, seek to increase it a little bit every week. Let go of perfectionist thinking that says, "It's not enough." Tell yourself instead that, "A little bit is better than nothing." Strive to build a life-long habit versus temporary spurts of activity followed by long gaps of inactivity. Forgive yourself for being less than perfect, and most importantly, don't give up.

The U.S. Department of Health and Human services outlines the following information about exercise in an article at www.healthierus.gov[4] :

Exercise:

- "Increases physical fitness.
- Helps build and maintain healthy bones, muscles, and joints.
- Builds endurance and muscular strength.
- Helps manage weight.
- Lowers risk factors for cardiovascular disease, colon cancer, and type-2 diabetes.
- Helps control blood pressure.

---

4   http://www.womenshealth.gov/faq/exercise.htm

- Promotes psychological well-being and self-esteem.
- Reduces feelings of depression and anxiety."

This same website article recommends: "Aim to accumulate at least 30 minutes (adults) or 60 minutes (children) of moderate physical activity most days of the week, preferably daily. If you already get 30 minutes of physical activity daily, you can gain even more health benefits by increasing the amount of time that you are physically active or by taking part in more vigorous activities. No matter what activity you choose, you can do it all at once, or spread it out over two or three times during the day." As you can see, the Donate Your Weight guidelines aren't as strict as the guidelines from the government. That's not because we disagree with the guidelines. Please aspire to meet this as a long-term goal. However, in my experience as a group leader, therapist and teacher, I have encountered hundreds of people who don't exercise at all. In fact, according to a 2005 report by the Center for Disease Control[5] regarding Trends in Leisure-Time Physical Inactivity, roughly 23% of all Americans are completely inactive. This means that millions of people are not exercising at all. If you're one of those people, please start where you are and strive to get better. The Donate Your Weight guidelines can be a stepping-stone to reaching the governmental guidelines. Chances are, as you begin to notice the benefits of exercise, you will want to do it more often simply because it makes your body feel good.

Strategy #5: Feed Your Mind, Change What You Say

This strategy is crucial to long-term, permanent weight-loss success. A research article in the *European Journal of Sport Science* (Annesi, James J., 2003), studied the relationship between using techniques such as "behavioral and cognitive behavioral treatments (e.g., goal setting, relapse prevention, self-reinforcement, contracting)" and the success rate of program participants. The research states that "Results of all 3 studies demonstrated significantly ($p < .05$) higher attendance (13–30%) and less drop out (30–39%) for the treatment groups, compared to their respective controls."

In street terms that means that when people used goal setting, rewards and techniques based on changing thinking and behavior, they were more successful in their exercise program and less likely to drop out. That's why at least half of this book is dedicated to helping you develop more positive skills such as improved self-talk, goal-setting, group support and behavior modification. Monitoring your thinking is just as important as monitoring your food intake,

---

5   http://www.cdc.gov/mmwr/preview/mmwrhtml/mm5439a5.htm

because when it comes right down to it, your thinking impacts your food and eating choices.

Let's take the example of two women, both working to improve their health and change their eating. We've got Successful Susie and Failing Frieda. Successful Susie's attention is on the positive. She admits it's a challenge to change habits, but she makes a conscious effort to focus most of her thoughts and energy on the benefits of improved health, energy, and appearance, rather than giving too much thought to the drawbacks of cutting down on some of her favorite foods and exercising regularly. Successful Susie knows this is a life-long process that she must incorporate into her life so she can have long-term results and fewer struggles with her weight and eating. Failing Frieda, on the other hand, is only focused on what she has to give up and what she can't have. She views her weight-loss attempt as something she has to temporarily endure until she eventually reaches her goal. She looks forward to the day when she can "cheat" again. Both Susie and Frieda are following their plan and taking the recommended steps. Which do you think will be most successful in achieving and maintaining results? The answer is clear: Successful Susie has the upper hand. Even though both of them are taking the same action, Frieda is already setting herself up for failure as she focuses on how boring the plan is and how much she can't wait to go back to eating unlimited potato chips every day.

The best news about this strategy is that we have a choice about whether we place our attention on the positive or the negative. You can choose to adopt Successful Susie's mentality, partially through simply setting your intention to do so, and partially with the help of the tools and techniques recommended in Chapters 4-6.

The bottom line is, you'll be more successful if you choose to focus on where you want to go than if you choose to focus on current struggles or struggles from the past. Focus on the positive aspects of making a long-term change, and regularly remind yourself of the benefits you'll experience from doing things a new way. Here's a partial list to get you started; fill in the blank spots with some of your own personal benefits from shifting your habits over the long term:

Benefits you'll achieve by developing a healthy lifestyle and healthy habits:
1. Release excess body weight
2. Have clothes fit better
3. Have more energy
4. Feel less joint pain
5. Lower cholesterol
6. Feel stronger

7.   Sleep better at night
8.   Enjoy health improvements
9.   Feel proud and confident
10.   Save money on junk food
11.   _____
12.   _____
13.   _____
14.   _____
15.   _____

Write out the items on this list that apply to you, make additions to the list as needed, and then carry it with you and review it daily as a part of the action plan you'll be developing in chapter 5.

Harnessing the Power of Affirmations

So many of us have learned to be our own worst enemies, but with practice, we can learn to be our own best friends. With a little dedication and commitment to yourself, you can begin chipping away at that low self-esteem and negativity and chiseling away that extra weight—thus uncovering the "lighter" you that hides within. Because your mind affects your body, what you say to yourself is as important as what you eat in determining your health and wellness. In this chapter, I will outline a comprehensive "mental diet" for your mind, so that you can regularly feed your mind healthy, positive affirmations that will support you in all of your efforts and allow you to achieve your goals.

Proper use of affirmations can be extremely powerful. However, casual reading of them will produce nothing more than a temporary boost in spirits, if that. So in order to get maximum benefit from this strategy, it's important to learn what an affirmation is and how to use it effectively.

My favorite definition of an affirmation is "the truth told in advance." When we firmly hold a belief, we tend to make it come true. It's called a self-fulfilling prophecy. We can take an active role in changing our beliefs and therefore create a new, more positive self-fulfilling prophecy.

While positive self-talk is only one component of a successful and permanent weight-loss program, it is a powerful, effective, no-cost tool that begins to help you shift your perspective and realize new possibilities. It's crucial that affirmations are repeated many times in order for them to slowly take the place of the negative self-talk we're used to having every day. Just like with effective advertising, it's important to remember that one "exposure" to a positive thought won't make an impact on your behavior; it's continued repetition that can make the behavioral change permanent.

Repetition and reinforcement are time-honored marketing principles that you can use to support yourself in achieving your goals. You don't need money or a degree or any special materials or tools. Only desire, persistence, and faith are needed, and you can be well on your way to creating lasting change.

Because it's easier for the mind to understand and remember small bits of information repeated over and over than large bits presented occasionally, choose between five and twenty affirmations from the following list to get started. More is not better. You will only overwhelm yourself if you try to work with more than twenty affirmations at a time. Along the same lines, once you choose your affirmations, work with the same ones over and over until you "get them," rather than changing them every week. Continue with the same affirmations over and over until it feels completely true for you or you make the change you have affirmed. Only after you've mastered your initial set of affirmations should you then choose a new set that reflects your changing goals. Don't get caught in the trap of impatience and wanting to change things continuously. The principles of persistence and patience are much more powerful than an endless string of new and constantly changing ideas.

Choosing from Sample Affirmations

As you review the following sample affirmations, read them s-l-o-w-l-y. Savor them. Pause between sentences (just like you pause between each bite). As you read them, ask yourself: How would my life/body be different if I believed this statement 100 percent, without reservation? What would I do differently? How would I feel?

Some of the affirmations will feel attainable to you, while others may feel, "Pie in the sky," or "Too good to be true." Choose those that feel believable, but stretch a little bit beyond your comfort zone. An affirmation should never be so far-fetched that you can't believe it's possible. The more you can imagine these statements as being true for you, the more likely you are to do what it takes to make them true.

Sometimes it feels especially good to hear someone else singing your praises. If you'd like to hear these affirmations come from someone else's voice other than your own, I have recorded several CD's you might find beneficial. These CD's and purchasing info are on the resource page in the back of this book. The benefit of using a CD or cassette tape to listen to your affirmations is that it's much easier to utilize the power of repetition with these recordings. With CD's, you can play a track and choose repeat mode so that the same track plays endlessly on your player. You can also do the same thing if you add your affirmation track to your mp3 player. You can use repeat mode to play the track over and over. This way, you can listen in your car or while you exercise, or even in the background as you work or clean the house. Here are some sample affirmations to get you started.

Expressing Self-Love

I love and appreciate my body, my mind, and my feelings.
I am nice to my body. I do what's best for it.
I love and accept my body as it is.
The more I love myself and others, the easier it is to lose weight.
I love my body enough to allow it to become thin and healthy.
I think positive thoughts about my body and encourage it to be the best it can be.
Because I love my body, I give it optimal treatment and allow it to become as healthy and vibrant as possible.
I am patient with myself, and I am going through changes at the perfect pace for me.
I love and accept my body right now.
Because I love my body, I only do what's best for it.

Feeling Gratitude

My body is inherently wise.
I am grateful for the life experiences that have brought me to this point.
My body is a miracle.
I show gratitude toward my body by treating it with respect and taking good care of it.
I trust my body.
My body is a miraculous gift.
I am thankful for my ears and all that I've been able to experience thanks to them.
I am grateful for my eyes and for my ability to read the words on this page.
I am grateful for my nose and my ability to smell various rich and sweet aromas.
I am grateful for the health I do have.
I am thankful that I am finally able to take care of myself the way I deserve.
I am grateful for my legs that carry me from place to place.
I am grateful for my arms that allow me to hold, carry and embrace many things in life.

Releasing Weight

I clear all emotional blocks and negative energy from my body; as a result, it functions beautifully.

I release all self-blame.

I release feelings that are bottled up inside me.

As I let go of repressed, heavy feelings, my body becomes lighter, thinner, and healthier.

I release perfectionist ideals of who I "should" be and accept myself as I am.

I let go of the past. I let go of the future. I am free to be me right now.

I relax and enjoy my life as it is which allows me to let go of my weight with greater ease.

My body functions efficiently and I give it optimal treatment to help it function even better.

I let go of the past. Today is a new day and I have a new attitude. Today I am a success.

Today I take all actions necessary to reach my goals.

I am patient with myself and I enjoy the process.

Acting "As If"

I keep a mental picture of my ideal body in the forefront of my mind.

I walk, talk, eat, breathe, and act like a person who has a healthy, thin, attractive body.

My habits are evolving and I'm becoming the thin, toned, healthy person I want to be.

I enjoy low-fat, high-fiber foods.

I enjoy fresh fruits and vegetables.

I notice the changes in how my clothes fit.

I love to feel toned, thin, and energetic.

I take good care of my body.

Making Positive Declarations

I maintain the right to decide what is attractive by my own standards.

No one else is exactly like me.

My body deserves to be treated with respect.

I deserve the good feelings that come with taking care of my body.

I'm becoming thinner and more attractive now.

I let go of the victim role and decide to be victorious instead.

I find solutions that empower me and make me a better person.

I refuse to allow someone else to determine the size and shape of my body.

I am in control of the size and shape of my body, and I now let go of excess, uncomfortable weight.

I am in control of my food choices.

I am in control of what I eat, when I eat, and how much I eat.

I eat the perfect amount for me.

I have tremendous inner-strength.

I like the way my body feels when it's light and thin.

Everything I do creates a better body for me.

I am excited about the positive changes that are taking place in my body right now.

I prefer a light, healthy feeling over a full, heavy feeling.

I always do the best I can.

I can trust myself.

I listen to my body.

Enhancing Your Metabolism

My metabolism is rapid and efficient.

My metabolism zooms.

My metabolism works day and night.

The food I eat burns up like logs in a fireplace.

I eat small amounts of food regularly, and my metabolism stays active day and night.

I eat slowly and chew my food thoroughly, which helps my metabolism work even better.

Food moves through my system and is metabolized rapidly.

Everything I eat is processed thoroughly and my body functions efficiently.

My metabolism is like a blazing fire that burns fuel quickly and efficiently.

Moving Your Body

I enjoy the benefits of regular activity.

I engage in physical exercise I enjoy.

I make plenty of time in my life for exercise.

I like the increased energy I feel when I exercise regularly.

I find that as I exercise more regularly, I sleep more soundly.

I create an environment that's conducive to regular exercise.

I use an exercise plan that fits my schedule.

I have an extra pep in my step when I exercise.

I exercise because I enjoy the benefits.

Exercise energizes my mind and body.

Setting Boundaries
I listen to and honor my feelings.
I surround myself with loving, good, positive feelings.
I trust my judgment.
I stand up for myself when something is uncomfortable.
I take care of myself.
I set an imaginary boundary around my body, and I decide who enters my personal space.
I let go of the past.
As I become thinner and healthier, my power to take care of myself increases.
There are better ways to protect myself than holding on to extra weight.
I learn to listen to myself.
I respect my needs.

Writing Personalized Affirmations
Using the pre-written affirmations above will provide you with a powerful starting point. Once you become familiar with the process of using affirmations daily, you might want to also practice writing your own personalized affirmations. Using a personalized affirmation has added benefits over using pre-written affirmations. Words are powerful and personal. Words like "thin, success, skinny, voluptuous, happy and joyful" mean different things to different people. Affirmations are most powerful when you use the words that are packed with positive and desirable associations that appeal to your own personality and long-term goals. A small change in wording can make a drastic change in impact. Remember the advertisers again, one word can literally make or break a successful campaign. When creating your affirmations, consider using power-packed words like exuberant, abundantly, soaring, tingly, exceptional, reveling in or basking in. Use words that excite you and that paint a mental picture you are able to see clearly. Use colors, shapes and scenes that you can imagine vividly. One of my workshop participants felt a particular glee when she affirmed and visualized seeing herself in a bikini in Jamaica. This was a very fun and pleasurable time in her life and remembering it made her feel positive and passionate about reaching her weight and body image goals.

Effective affirmations are:
- Written in the present tense as if they are true now
- Clear statements of what you want. (Avoid affirmations that mention the condition you are trying to change. Keep your focus on where you want to go)
- Specific, vivid, lively, awe-inspiring, emotion provoking

■   Visual. It's almost like you can see, feel or touch them

Here's a sample framework for affirmation writing. Play around with it until you find what fits. "I _____ (insert your name here), am _____ _____ (insert an exciting, fun word here) moving toward _____ __ (insert specific goal here) with _____ (insert emotion here). I can see myself _____ (insert words to describe image here) now. I achieve _____ (insert specific goal here) with ease and grace."

Techniques for Effective Use of Affirmations

Now that you're familiar with affirmations, I want to share four techniques I recommend: affirmation cards, endless cassettes or CDs, affirmation journal, and affirmations with an anchor. The reason you'll want to choose one of these techniques is that they all use the power of repetition which will make or break your success with affirmations. Affirmations are like commercials. The more often you experience them in your day-to-day life, the more likely they are to influence you. Choose the technique that feels best to you, or use a combination of these techniques. Do at least one of these techniques daily.

Affirmation Technique #1: Affirmation Cards

Choose five to twenty affirmations that you really want to concentrate on. Put each affirmation on its own card, and make a point to review the cards several times daily. You may want to put these on your bedside table, so you can review them in the morning before you get out of bed and before you go to sleep. In order to get maximum benefit, use colorful cards and colorful markers. If you're artistic, draw little pictures on your cards. If not, use stickers to liven them up. You can also purchase colorful, artistically designed affirmation cards such as those listed on the resource page.

Affirmation Technique #2: Endless Affirmations

Especially if you tend to learn better through hearing something than seeing it, you may want to listen to recordings of your affirmations. You can either purchase an endless-loop cassette tape and record your affirmations on that, record your affirmations on a CD or mp3 and listen to them on repeat mode, or buy an affirmation CD that you can listen to throughout your day. (See resource page for details).

Affirmation Technique #3: Affirmation Journal

You can use an affirmation journal to write down the five to twenty affirmations you want to work with, and then spend fifteen to thirty minutes each day rewriting them in that journal. Repeatedly writing your affirmations out puts the power of repetition in your favor. As you write in the journal you are reading, seeing, saying, and feeling your affirmations over and over again. The repetition helps the affirmations feel more natural to you, so that when good things start coming into your life, you will be mentally prepared to handle them and enjoy them.

Affirmation Technique #4: Affirmations with an Anchor

In this technique, you choose an anchor, such as a smooth rock, marble or piece of jewelry that you can rub as you say your affirmations. Repeating your affirmations aloud or silently while rubbing the anchor will help build an association between the anchor and affirmations. With repeated practice, you can soon rub the anchor and it will remind you of your affirmations. This way, you can "bring along" your affirmations throughout your day by simply touching your anchor when you need to remember them most. (Donate Your Weight offers a Slim Image Power Pack complete with affirmation cards, anchors and mini-instruction booklet. See the Resource Page for details.)

Avoiding the Potential Pitfalls of Affirmations

As fantastic and effective as affirmations can be, there are some potential pitfalls that can impede their progress. Staying aware of these potential pitfalls can help ensure that your affirmations are working for you optimally.

Possible Pitfall #1: Acting as a Tenant Rather than an Owner

In Fredric Lehrman's audio program *Prosperity Consciousness* (Nightingale Conant 1992), he suggests that we remember that our current line of thinking has been rehearsed and nurtured for many, many years, and that the part of our personality that feels content with the "comfortable" way of being isn't going to change easily.

He then asks us to imagine that our various negative beliefs are tenants in the apartment building of our minds. These tenants have lived here a long time and feel pretty comfortable with things "just the way they are." Suddenly, we come along with an announcement: "I'm going to make things better. Fix broken pipes, paint the walls, even put in new carpet." The tenants begin to perk up at the prospect of this positive change until you announce that you will also be raising the rent. "*What!?!!*" they respond, "You're going to *what!?!!*" The part about carpet and paint sounded great, but once you mention a rent increase, the tenants will probably say, "Things are just fine the way they are," "Why change things now?" or, "I can't afford it."

You might be surprised to hear that this "tenant reaction" is a natural and automatic reaction to change. Don't be alarmed or judge your reaction. Simply observe. If your mind begins to freak out when you start doing positive affirmations, remember one thing: *you* are the owner! It's up to you to stick to your guns, be persistent, and stick to the plan. The tenants will thank you later. Trust me.

Possible Pitfall #2: Magical Thinking

Affirmations can be powerful. Sometimes you begin noticing changes almost immediately. It's tempting to take this newfound power and run wild with it. You might start thinking, "Oh cool, all I have to do is say, 'I am skinny,' for thirty days and I'll be skinny." Okay, maybe you will become slimmer but it won't happen simply because you say it will.

Affirmations are intended to facilitate a mindset that leads to positive actions; you have to take actions that coincide with your affirmations to get results. Don't get trapped into thinking that affirmations alone will solve all your problems. You have to combine positive self-talk with positive action, and apply a heavy dose of consistency and patience to that mix. Permanent change doesn't happen overnight. Look at nature for examples: A rose bush has full potential to be beautiful, strong, and productive from the moment it's planted. However, if it isn't provided with the proper nutrients and environmental elements, consistently and over time the end result may be long, spindly, weak stems with loosely formed buds that fall apart quickly. That's not to say it isn't beautiful in its own way, but it hasn't reached its full potential. If that same rosebush is nurtured and given the correct environmental needs, over a period of time it will be stronger, more vibrant, and more productive.

The same is true with you. Yes, you might get results right away, but that doesn't mean it's time to take off and forget all about the process that leads to permanent results. Don't think you've "arrived" just because you see a bit of change taking place. Instead, if you want to witness continual, steady, strong, permanent and lasting change, you must stay the course.

Possible Pitfall #3: Cover-Up Affirmations

Because affirmations are positive and life-affirming and sometimes make us feel so darn good, it's tempting to use them as a sort of bandage for hurt, disappointment, shame, regret, etc. You are misusing affirmations when you try to pretend you feel or think something that you don't really feel or think.

For example, if you're depressed and you tell yourself, "I am happy" over and over, and pretend to be happy even though you feel miserable, you won't get the help you need and the situation can actually get worse. Affirmations aren't meant to be used to lie about something or pretend that something doesn't exist. However, affirmations can help you to get a broader perspective because you are focusing on numerous possibilities versus focusing only on the negative. It is 100 percent true that change is possible and that you can change your negative beliefs and counterproductive behaviors. It is also important to honor yourself where you are in this moment, so you can learn more about yourself and identify what needs to be examined or tended to in your life. If you deny problems or challenges, you lose power and energy because it takes effort to push those uncomfortable thoughts and feelings away. On the other hand, if you tend to these issues as they come up, they actually lose power. As a result, when you meet challenges straight on and tackle them, you have more energy to create the life you want.

Strategy #6: Do Self-Hypnosis Every Day

As we've already discussed, what you think and say greatly impacts your behaviors and your degree of success. So just as it's important to feed your body healthy foods every day, it's imperative to your success to feed your mind healthy thoughts and ideas every day. In this section, you'll learn the many ways you can utilize self-hypnosis as a positive tool for change.

Doing Daily Self-Hypnosis

There are a lot of unfortunate misconceptions about hypnosis because of exaggerated depictions in TV and movies of people being hypnotized into doing something wild, crazy, and out of their control. In actuality, hypnosis is a relaxation technique that helps you turn down the volume on the critical mind so you can access your creative, subconscious mind and do the very things you really want to do with greater ease.

Hypnosis can't make you do anything against your will. It's important to note that in stage hypnosis shows, the hypnotist chooses *volunteers* from the audience—people who, for whatever reason, want to be hypnotized on a stage. Then the hypnotist performs a series of tests to be sure the volunteer is really a good, willing subject, and that they didn't just volunteer so they could prove they were unable to be hypnotized. The volunteers who fail to pass a few susceptibility tests are guided off the stage and back to their seats. By the time the show begins, the stage is filled with willing, susceptible people who want to be hypnotized on a stage. These "cast members" are likely extroverted and enjoy doing crazy things to make people laugh, which is why the hypnotists are able to get them to cluck like chickens or do other silly or embarrassing things.

Stage hypnosis is quite different from the experience of self-hypnosis. By the way, it is called self-hypnosis because you will only be in a state of hypnosis if you choose to be, it is not something that can happen entirely against you will. You can access the power of hypnosis by using recordings or by working with a professionally trained hypnotherapist. In each case, the hypnotherapist will guide you through a series of relaxation techniques that can help you be more susceptible to specific positive thoughts that will enhance your success in your related goals.

With practice and determination, you can also do this relaxation process on your own. You simply have to be willing to take the time and to let go of your habitual conscious thoughts that stand between you and the slimmer, healthier body you desire. Allowing yourself to relax completely enables you to shut off the conscious, critical mind that has likely been getting in the way of your success.

For example, your conscious mind might be filled with critical thoughts such as, "You can't lose weight now, what about the kids?," "Oh, not another diet, you won't get to eat any of the things you like and it will be boring," or "If you lose weight, you'll need all new clothes, and you can't afford it." You can turn down the volume on these thoughts and replace them with more positive beliefs that will support rather than sabotage your success.

Although there may be some truth to what the conscious, critical mind says, if you listen to it and believe everything it says 100 percent, you'll stay stuck and continue repeating the same patterns and getting the same results. Hypnosis helps you get the conscious mind out of the way so you can access your subconscious mind, which is much more open to change and possibility. Your subconscious mind controls your habits and behaviors. When you access your subconscious mind in a relaxed state, you access that part of you that "dares to dream." Your subconscious mind is not hung up on being right, and it's completely open to suggestion and willing to try new things. If you are able to relax enough to talk to your subconscious mind, you can get this power in your corner and achieve tremendous results.

Here's how a typical self-hypnosis session goes:

1. Get really, really relaxed but don't fall asleep.
2. Imagine yourself successfully working toward and achieving your goal. Imagine the process in rich detail. Tell yourself what you're going to do, and see yourself doing it.

3. "Wake up" from the experience feeling energized and optimistic. Now that your subconscious mind knows what you really want to achieve, it can help you in finding ways to accomplish what you said you wanted to accomplish.

There are several approaches to self-hypnosis. You can use hypnosis CDs, visit a hypnotherapist in his or her office, or, with practice, learn self-hypnosis techniques you can use yourself. If you decide to learn self-hypnosis, recognize that it will take practice and that you will have to trust that it is working in the beginning, even when it feels like it's not. When you first get started, it can help to buy a prerecorded CD that supports long-term, permanent weight loss, such as the ones listed at the back of this book. In the meantime, you can use the following self-hypnosis technique so you can get started today. Set aside at least 15-20 minutes to incorporate the following the steps of self-hypnosis 3–7 times per week.

Step 1: Relax

There are many ways to do this; here are a few suggestions so you can choose whatever works for you. Since relaxation sets the stage for a receptive mind, this step is very important and will probably take the most time. Spend as much as 7-15 minutes just relaxing your mind and body.

1. Take deep, slow, rhythmic breaths, breathing slower and slower as time progresses.
2. Imagine that the breath you inhale is a mellow, relaxing color and the breath you exhale is a color representing stress, tension, and/or negativity. Breathe in calm, breathe out tension.
3. Focus on a pleasing, relaxing object such as a candle flame, the water flowing from a fountain, or the trees blowing in the breeze. Fix your concentration on this image until you begin to feel carefree and dreamlike. Close your eyes to deepen the relaxation and imagine your eyelids getting heavy.
4. Imagine a time when you were very relaxed (for instance, after a massage, on vacation, after you fell asleep on the couch, sitting in a hot tub, etc.). Imagine this physical experience so vividly that you begin to relive it in your mind and body.

Step 2: Imagine What You Want

Spend five to eight minutes to imagine what you want in very vivid detail. Focus only on what you want to be (not on what you don't want). For example, if you want to stop overeating at night, imagine yourself having an evening free from overeating. See yourself eating small amounts or avoiding food all together. Imagine feeling peaceful about this and accomplishing it with ease. Or, if you want to be more consistent with exercise, imagine yourself exercising and really enjoying it. See yourself accomplishing the goals you've set for yourself. Add detail to the imagery. Imagine wearing a color and size that you feel positive about. Imagine your body posture being confident and proud, just like you'd feel if you already achieved your goal. Add as much rich detail to this time period as possible. See yourself wearing your favorite clothes and feeling comfortable and confident in your own skin.

Step 3: Wake Up

It's helpful to have a phrase to help you become fully alert after your session is complete. You can count from one to five slowly, or say, "When I open my eyes, I'll be wide awake, refreshed, and ready to tackle my day." You can also twitch your finger or rotate your ankles to help you get back in touch with the current moment. This step only takes about 15-60 seconds. Be sure to sit still for a few moments after you open your eyes. Give your body time to adjust before you bolt up and get back to business.

Help, I don't have time!

These words are often used as a reason not to integrate self-care into your day. But the truth is, if you watch TV, drive a car, surf the internet, or listen to the radio, you are being hypnotized daily. Advertisers and marketers have spent years of time, hours of research, and billions of dollars to bring you the best of all hypnotic techniques delivered directly to your monitor and speakers every day. Why not steal back some of that time and use it to implement your own pre-chosen programming for goal achievement. It beats being an unconscious recipient of someone else's programming. Here are some fun and creative ways to do that.

1.   Reassess your TV menu. Cut out one show you can live without and replace it with a self-hypnosis session.
2.   Notice the commercials and ads that really draw you in. Is it the flashing screen that renders you motionless? Or is it the cute songs that you can't resist singing to? Maybe it's the imagery that draws you in? Study the ads that really pull you in and do the following with your newfound information:
      a) Create an ad of your own that utilizes the elements that impact you most; for example, maybe your own affirmation song or jingle.

b) If the flickering screen pulls you in, use a flickering candle or even a video of flickering flames to help you get into the hypnotic state.

c) If you love the images in ads, create your own images, or cut and paste images from magazines, remembering to choose positive and realistic images.

One of the reasons billboard advertising has such a powerful impact is that many drivers are in a hypnotic state when they see these images. How many times have you found yourself arriving at work or home and not remembering how you got there? If that has happened to you, it's because you were in a hypnotic state. Another example of driving while hypnotized is when you get off at an exit you hadn't intended to get off at. For example, you might get in the car and consciously decide to get off at a different exit or take a different route on the way home so you can run an errand. If you're like most people, you've had at least one or two instances where you habitually got off at the exit you always get off at rather than taking the alternate route you had consciously set out to take.

So, now that you know you're already being hypnotized every day, use it to your benefit. The following tips will help you to use your hypnotic time wisely and find ways to make time for self-hypnosis sessions.

Post colorful affirmations in your car. Look at them instead of the billboards.

Create your own jingles to go along with highly powerful advertisements. Turn down the volume and sing your own version.

Cut out one of the shows you watch and do self-hypnosis instead.

Tape your favorite shows or get Tivo. Fast forward through the commercials and use the extra time to do your self-hypnosis.

Do self-hypnosis first thing in the morning so you won't have to worry about squeezing it in later.

Put colorful affirmations and positive pictures near your computer so you always have positive images and thoughts surrounding you. These images will become stronger than any advertisement could ever be because: a) the images are chosen by you and personally powerful to you and b) you are exposed to them for hours and hours each day whereas you are only exposed to advertisements in brief, fleeting and random flashes.

Listen to affirmations or positive books on tape in the car. If you're hypnotized anyway, might as well use the time to your advantage!

Strategy #7: Pamper Yourself, Don't Delay

What does pampering have to do with weight loss, you ask? Well, for many of us food has become the primary "treat" or "reward" we allow ourselves when we feel sad, mad, celebratory, insecure, glad, bored, restless, anxious, and so on. So in order to give up eating as a reward, we need to find a multitude of alternative ways to be nice to ourselves and "treat" ourselves. Food is supposed to be fuel for our bodies, not a "cure" for a broken heart or job stress. And ultimately, there are much more satisfying and healthy ways to find soothing and happiness.

In many cases, we have become so busy taking care of others that we put ourselves last. This sets up a cycle that frequently leads to overeating. We eat to comfort ourselves and to reward ourselves as a compensation for not taking care of ourselves in other areas of life. Figure 4.1 demonstrates how when we "over-do" it can often lead to exhaustion, stress, hurt and feelings of self-neglect. These feelings are often the driving force behind late night binges.

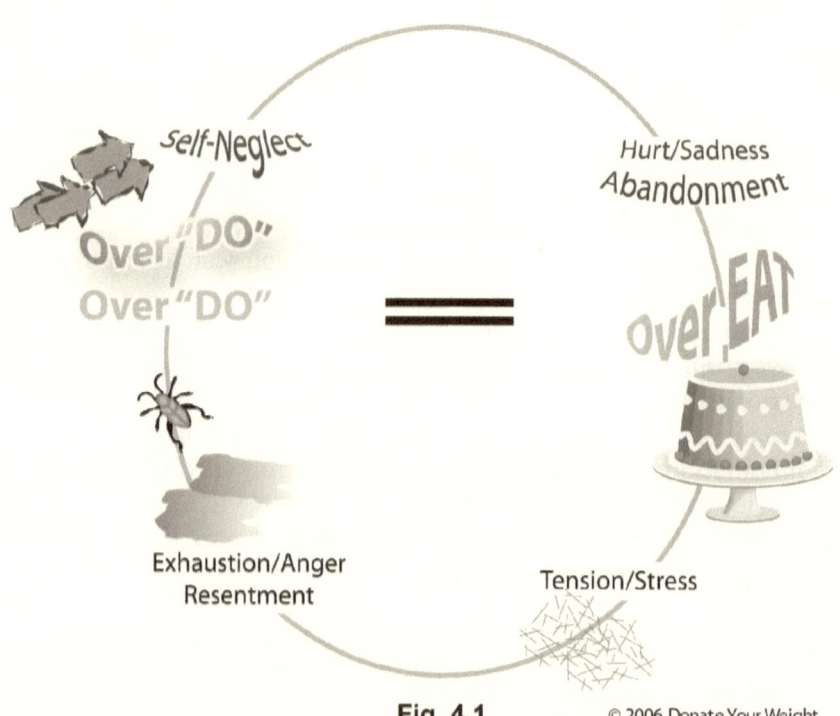

Fig. 4.1   © 2006 Donate Your Weight

When we begin to take time for ourselves and to practice regular self-care, we can break the cycle of comfort eating.

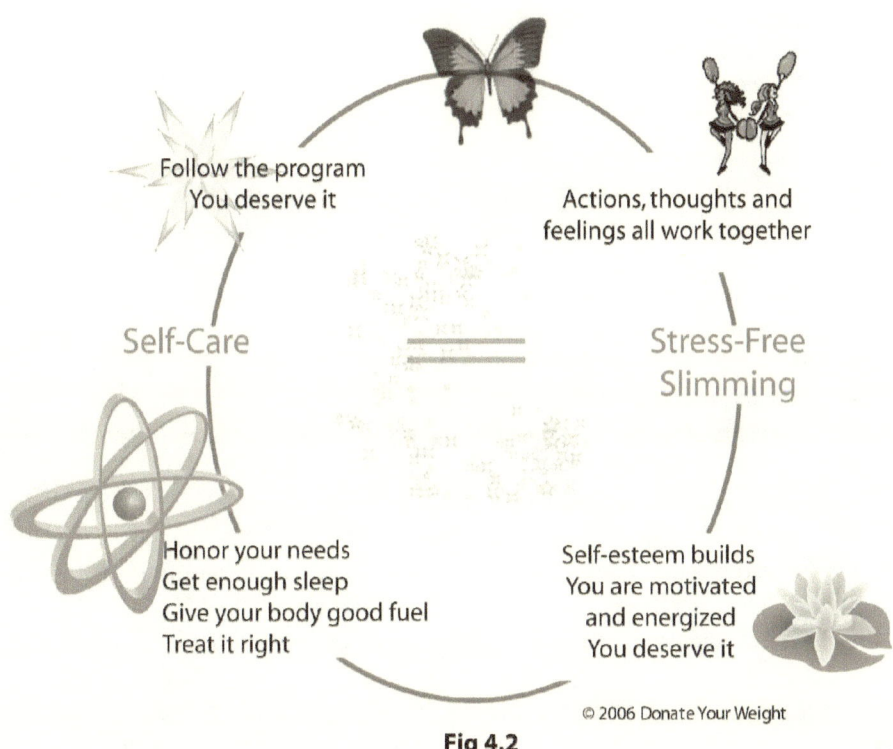

Fig 4.2

The following list is just a small sampling of ways you can reward or treat yourself:

- Take a bubble bath
- Get a manicure or pedicure
- Watch your favorite movie or TV show
- Go for a walk on the beach or another beautiful place
- Give yourself a foot massage
- Read a good book or magazine
- Go to a museum
- Light a scented candle and relax on the couch
- Sip some warm herbal tea

- Listen to soothing or uplifting music
- Look at a book with beautiful images
- Dance in your living room or out at a club
- Write all of your deepest dreams and fears in your journal
- Compose a poem or song
- Draw or paint
- Rearrange your living space
- Knit a scarf
- Go to a concert
- Do a jigsaw puzzle, crossword puzzle, or other game
- Play a board game by yourself or with friends
- Garden
- Buy fresh flowers
- Spend the day in a nearby town you don't know well
- Go somewhere and people watch
- Go to an amusement park or county fair
- Call someone you really want to talk to, even if it's long distance
- Change your hair or your make-up for a "new look"
- Give yourself a home facial
- Take a fun class
- Go to a sporting event, a play, a reading, or a comedy show
- Take a long drive
- Go on a pleasurable walk or hike, or ride a bike someplace in nature

Some of the items on this list will probably appeal to you more than others. Choose a few you feel genuinely excited about and use them to help you get started with pampering yourself. This is an opportunity for you to make it a priority to begin putting yourself first more often and start treating yourself the way you would treat someone you love very much.

Modifying the Seven Slimming Strategies for Children

If you are raising a child or adolescent, a variation of these seven steps can also help you raise children who get regular activity, eat healthily, and think positively. It's never too late to make a change and support your child's health in a positive, affirming way. Here are some suggestions:

- Reevaluate portions: Our stomachs are about the size of our fists, so remember to give your children portions that are the sizes of their fists, not yours.

- Never force them to "finish everything on their plates." Instead, help them learn healthy eating by presenting them with reasonable portions of nutritious foods. Model the behavior of saving leftovers. Teach them to choose appropriate portions. Require them to eat a little bit of each item on the plate and encourage a balanced and healthy way of eating.

- Limit most snacks to either leftovers from meals or small, single servings of healthier foods like fruit, nuts, and cheese and crackers. Entire bowls of cereal and sandwiches are more like a meal than a snack, and should be saved for mealtimes. To avoid setting up feelings of deprivation or a sense of "bad" food, consider offering your child a choice of one of their favorite snack foods several times a week, in a fist-sized portion.

- Lead by example. Children pay more attention to what you do than what you say. If you want to spare your child from weight and eating obsession and body image distortions, begin by making a commitment to change yourself. Children are incredibly perceptive and intuitive. If you worry about your weight, they will worry about their weight. Decide today to be a role model of healthy habits and a realistic body image.

- Exercise with your children. Try to make exercise a regular family activity, such as after-school or after-dinner walks or bike rides.

- Replace fear with facts. Check with a doctor or other relatives before automatically assuming that drastic changes in diet are necessary. You may discover that your child's temporary changes in size/shape are a normal and temporary part of the growing process. Don't apply unrealistic ideals to your child's body.

- Feed their minds. You can use affirmations with your child by simply repeating positive phrases to them all the time in your daily reactions. Focus on their successes, praise them for drinking water, getting exercise, and knowing when they're finished eating. As adults, we use affirmations to counter negative thoughts and ideas that often started when we were children ourselves. We can help lay a groundwork of high self-esteem for our children by teaching them positive ways to soothe themselves and express their feelings (rather than eating for comfort) and offering them affirming statements on a daily basis, like, "I believe in you," "You're doing a great job," "I'm so proud of you," and "I love you." If you still find yourself criticizing more than praising your child, it's a positive indicator that maybe its time for the whole family to seek help.

- Teach children to bite, chew, swallow, pause, and teach them that it's okay to leave food on their plate.
- Offer them plenty of water to drink (you can add orange slices for flavor if that's helpful).
- Recognize each of their positive steps, and consider offering them a sticker for each time they eat slowly, get exercise, etc. Consider starting a graduated point system and helping them come up with a reasonable list of their own rewards, such as staying up ten minutes past bedtime, days in the park, cuddle time with you on the couch, watching a favorite video, getting to play their favorite video game as much as they want on a weekend day, etc.
- Play a positive CD for them as they drift off to sleep. Some mothers play the *Love Your Body, Love Yourself* CD for their children at night. They mention that their children respond well and fall to sleep quickly. This CD is about self-love and honoring your body and can be helpful for all ages and sizes. (See resources page for details.)

A Note about Nutrition

You may have noticed that I haven't included a food plan yet. I haven't told you what to eat. This is probably quite different than what you're used to. Well, first off, I'm not a nutritionist so I'm not going to try and dispense nutritional information here. Secondly, it has been my experience that dieters know a lot about nutrition. Yet, all the nutritional information in the world has done little to help any of us solve our weight problem. The Donate Your Weight program agrees with an Intuitive Eating approach as outlined in a book of the same name by authors Evelyn Tribole and Elyse Resch (who are, by the way, nutritionists.) If you are deeply concerned about nutrition, consult a nutritional expert or seek out unbiased, research-based information about food and how it impacts your body. Many times food and nutrition information that is provided by weight loss programs is misleading or incomplete. Strive to find information that will improve your health and the weight reduction will follow. Seek out professional advice that honors your culture, your age, and your individual needs Avoid a cookie-cutter plan that may or may not be healthy or livable for you.

CHAPTER 5

DONATE YOUR WEIGHT

This chapter will answer the question you've probably been asking since you decided to buy this program: "How do I donate my weight?" No, you can't cut it off and send it to us but you can discover a way to free yourself from it for good. Read on and learn:

1) How to use the Donate Your Weight program with a group or organization to stop weight and eating struggles and help starving children at the same time.

2) How to use the Donate Your Weight program on an individual basis to stop weight and eating struggles while using the reward system to help you stay on track and focused on success.

Before I begin outlining the steps to start your Donate Your Weight program, I'd like to explain the Donate Your Weight reward plan. The reward plan is one of the motivating forces that will lead to great success whether you choose to work as a group or as an individual.

Focusing on Rewards is the Key to Success

Years of behavior modification research proves that focusing on desired behavior by tracking it and rewarding it leads to an increase in such behavior. One of the best ways to successfully change a habit is to track your desired behaviors and reward yourself each time you do things in the new and improved way. Rewards create an incentive and give you something to look forward to. When you focus on rewards, it's easier to follow through on what needs to be done.

The power of the Donate Your Weight program lies in focusing on rewards and fun versus deprivation and boredom. In Chapter four you learned the Seven Stress-Free Slimming Strategies. In this chapter, you'll learn to track your positive behavior and reward yourself for each success along the way.

The Donate Your Weight reward plan consists of utilizing the Success *Check*-list at the end of this book in conjunction with a reward bank. You are encouraged to use your Success *Check*-list all throughout the day to track your progress. Then, at the end of the evening you'll deposit money into your bank based on the successes you achieved during the day. This practice helps you to keep your focus on successes and off of temporary setbacks. Using a reward bank with real money creates a positive experience where you feel drawn to follow through on your desired behaviors because of the rewards attached. The subconscious mind controls much of your behavior and it loves games and rewards. Using the reward bank can distract you from the trials and challenges of self-change because your energy has shifted and now you're looking forward to the rewards of sticking to your plan instead of thinking about what you're missing out on by changing your behavior.

Many of us have been motivated by rewards since early childhood. As a result, rewards continue to drive our behavior in adulthood. In kindergarten we earned stickers, ribbons and candy for good behavior. In grade school we won awards, trophies and contests. Employers know that rewards can motivate employees to increase productivity and marketers use rewards to impact buying behavior. Billions of dollars in research and testing show that rewards work when it comes to creating behavior change. Using a reward plan in conjunction with the Seven Stress-Free Slimming Strategies helps you to garner the strength of your subconscious mind and get the power of your conscious and subconscious mind working together as a team rather than fighting against each other.

Using a reward system can also help you to break free from feelings of defeat and overwhelm. Many times we feel defeated by our weight-loss efforts before we start because we have had years of experience with temporary weight loss followed by the defeating and deflating experience of rapid and inevitable weight gain. In order to have permanent, lasting, life-long results, we will have to make some challenging behavior changes and endure some sacrifices. The evidence or manifestation of our efforts can take weeks, months, and even years to fully realize. Tracking your success on the *Check*-list and paying yourself money for success on a daily basis allows you to focus on the process rather than the end goal and to feel positive and successful all along the road to personal achievement and weight reduction.

Using the reward system helps you to feel positive every day, regardless of a number on the scale. As you institute the Stress-Free Slimming Strategies into your everyday life to the best of your ability, your feelings of confidence and self-control will increase. You will become aware of how each small change is an important part of the process. As you progress through the program and stick to it, you will also experience an abundance of real-life rewards such as stress-reduction, a feeling of self-control, pride, satisfaction, changes in habits and patterns, weight loss and more.

Collect Your Checks and Put Money in Your Bank

The best way to ensure your success with all the techniques mentioned in this book is to create a plan of action that prepares you to take the time necessary to incorporate these Strategies into your daily life. Ideally, you'll want to wake up each morning knowing exactly what your self-care goals are for the day so you'll be prepared mentally, emotionally and physically to succeed in following your plan. Try not to think of this as a short-term plan, but rather as a plan that you will use in some form (with adjustments for variety, of course), for your lifetime. It's important that you find ways to incorporate these Strategies into your life in a smooth, natural and automatic way.

It takes time, persistence, and patience to create new habits. Change doesn't happen by accident and it doesn't usually happen overnight. Remember, you didn't develop your current habits overnight and you probably won't create new habits overnight either. In fact, the definition of a habit is to do something over and over again until it becomes a natural part of your life. Now is your opportunity to commit to yourself how dedicated you will be. The first step is creating a daily action plan or schedule that makes it possible to incorporate the new techniques and habits you've learned about into your daily life. This might require some fine-tuning of your schedule and some prioritizing. It might require you to set firm boundaries for yourself and to be strong when others test your boundaries.

When things get tough, just remember why this is important to you. Remind yourself of the mental and emotional freedoms you'll gain when you can live free from excess weight. Imagine a life free from dieting, feeling deprived, depressed and "not good enough." The success and freedom you crave is possible but it's up to you to take the necessary steps and to stick with them until they become automatic. You can achieve the results you desire one step at a time.

Sample list of daily action steps and time required

Following is a quick reminder of all the things you'll want to include on your action plan and an estimated amount of time it will take to successfully accomplish all aspects of the program each day.

__ Review affirmations or listen to positive affirmation track (five minutes before I get out of bed)

__ Bite, chew, swallow, wait (with each meal *and* wait 3-5 hours between each meal)

__ Leave some food on my plate (with each meal)

__ Drink 48 ounces of water (start early in the day for best results)

__ Walk briskly while listening to affirmations recording (twenty minutes)

__ Listen to affirmation track in my car or while I do errands

__ Pamper myself with a treat from my rewards list (time varies 5 minutes to 2 hours)

__ Look at Beneficial Billboard or Self-Fulfilling Scrapbook (ten minutes before bed)

__ Tally my *Checks* and put money in my reward bank (five minutes)

__ Listen to self-hypnosis CD (20-30 minutes)

Your total time necessary to succeed at this program is about 75 minutes a day, plus conscious mealtimes, flexible time for weekly pampering and time for weekly support group meeting (60-90 minutes.)

Remember, this is a sample beginners plan and you can modify it to fit your needs. However, strive to incorporate all of most of the Strategies into your life on a daily basis. As you become comfortable, you can continue to increase the level of physical activity every couple of months, as your body gets used to it, until you're exercising for twenty minutes five times each week.

You can use the Donate Your Weight *Check*-list to track your successes all day long. Print out numerous copies so you have a new one for each week. In the evening, tally your successes for the day and place your reward in the reward bank. This way, you'll be tracking and acknowledging your successes in two ways: 1) in writing, and 2) with a monetary reward, this double reinforcement makes it that much more likely that you will continue to stay on track and experience on-going success. To make the reward process even more powerful, use a see-through bank so you can watch the money increase in your bank as you add to it each night. Also, put your bank some place where you are likely to see it numerous times each day so that you are subconsciously reinforcing your success many times per day.

Now that you have an idea of the time required to follow all aspects of the program, strategize ways to make it fit with your own existing schedule. If your original plan doesn't work, don't worry. Keep modifying until it fits. Focus on progress not perfection. Change can feel challenging at first, but remember that you're building a routine for a lifetime of good health, vibrant energy, and permanent weight maintenance. If you struggle with dedicating an hour or so every day to your self-care, make sure to read the section in the next chapter called, "Detour #2: Admit That You're Worth Taking the Time." Because even if you don't believe you have the time, your health is most definitely worth being a top priority! If you fail to make time for your health now, you may be forced to take time for it later in a much less enjoyable way.

If you're a frequent traveler, you will also need to figure out how you can incorporate your action plan into your trips. Many travelers with a diet history have "special" rules for eating/drinking behavior while they're away from home. They allow themselves to "go off" the diet or food plan and tell themselves, "I'll go back to being 'good' when I get home." If you travel more than once or twice a year, you'll need to reassess your attitudes about travel behavior. Remember, this isn't all about "feast or famine" or "all or nothing." For long-term, consistent results, weave these behaviors into your entire life, every day, whether you're at home or out of town.

Choosing a Reward Amount

Now that you're beginning to understand the reward concept and how it can help you change habits, you'll want to take time to consider your donation amount for each success. Since you'll be adding to your reward bank often and over a long period of time, it's important to choose an amount that goes with your budget. You'll never want to put yourself in a position where you can't afford the reward. This can lead to discouragement and defeat. It's important to reward yourself every time you do the new behavior and to use the money you collect for the specific purpose you'll decide on before starting the reward plan. Think about it, this concept is already working in your life right now. You go to work because you want a paycheck. Imagine what would happen if your employer stopped paying you. Would you still be motivated to go to work each day? Probably not. So again, please choose an amount that you can comfortably afford to maintain and that will inspire you to follow through with the behavior changes you desire to make.

The subconscious part of your mind is very childlike. If you break promises to yourself or set expectations of a reward that never comes, your subconscious mind will think, "What's the point of trying?" When that childlike part of yourself helps fuel your motivation to exercise and eat well with the expectation of a reward and you don't deliver, the mind won't believe your next promise and won't be as motivated to do the required steps to succeed. However, if you do follow through with the reward, the childlike part of you thinks, "Yippee, this is fun! I like helping out when it comes with all of these great rewards." As a result, this part of you feels genuinely excited to take the next step so it can get the next reward.

Consider this: if you eat three times a day and follow the program perfectly, you will earn approximately 25 *Checks* each day. So, choose a monetary amount that you can comfortably afford. Keep the following numbers in mind:

Daily Reward Amount	Weekly Total (x7)	Monthly Total (x30)
.01 x 25 = .25	1.75	7.50
.05 x 25 = 1.25	8.75	37.50
.10 x 25 = 2.50	17.50	75.00
.25 x 25 = 6.25	43.75	187.50

If some of the Strategies are extremely challenging for you, you might want to consider modifying your reward plan so that you get higher rewards for more difficult behaviors. In their book, *Self Directed Behavior*, professors David L. Watson and Roland G. Tharp (1993, 2006) suggest that rewards have some correlation to the difficulty of the behavior you are trying to establish. They also suggest that as the behavior becomes easier, the reward amount should decrease. The philosophy is that as the behaviors become part of your life, being slimmer and healthier becomes your primary reward. With these points in mind, here are some recommendations that might work for you.

- If one of the Strategies is much more difficult for you than the others, consider a double or even triple reward for the difficult behavior until it becomes easier.
- Decrease the reward as the behavior gets easier and easier.
- If strategy #3 (Drink Your Water 6x8) is very difficult for you, increase the reward with each 8 ounce glass. In other words, the first glass = 1 point, the second glasses = 2 points (for a total of 3 vs. 2) and so on.
- Be creative and flexible regarding all strategies. Find a way to stay motivated and break habits. Make your own rules for life.

Use Your *Check*-list and Reward Bank to Overcome Emotional/ Habit Hunger

Your *Check*-list has room for you to outline three goals of your own. You can use these extra spaces to target specific behaviors you'd like to overcome. Some examples might include, not eating after 7:00 p.m. or bypassing a habitual stop at your favorite fast food restaurant. Sometimes we have habits and rituals that have been around a long time. Using the *Check*-list and reward bank can help us to change these habits.

Sheila was well aware of the financial costs associated with emotional and habit eating and she decided to use her reward bank to overcome a fast food addiction while also donating money to help starving children in Africa. She knew that each trip to her favorite fast food restaurant cost roughly $3–5 so, each time she successfully avoided eating fast food on impulse, she put $3 in her reward bank. Sheila made a commitment to donate all her reward money to CARE via www.donateyourweight.org. Each time Sheila resisted the temptation to eat at her favorite fast food restaurant she was able to donate money to CARE and she felt satisfied that her money was going to a good cause.

Making this choice benefited Sheila in numerous ways. She was breaking free from her fast food addiction, she was helping others, she felt proud of herself and this impacted her life in many ways, she wasn't losing any money because she would have spent it anyway only now the money was going to something she felt good about. In reality, Sheila actually saved money because instead of spending $3–5 for each fast food trip she was only donating $3 plus, every time she resisted the temptation to eat emotionally she felt stronger and also avoided unnecessary excess calories that might have led to weight gain. Perhaps this tactic will work for you. Whether or not you follow this exact tactic, consider the fact that emotional eating and habit eating does cost money. Consider how much you can save if you don't eat emotionally and take this into consideration when choosing a donation amount for the week.

Once you've chosen your reward amount, you're ready to follow these steps and get started:

1. Create a reward bank for yourself. Use a clear jar or container so you can watch the rewards grow or use a coffee can embellished with pictures that represent reaching your goal. Make a hole in the lid so you can easily insert coins or folded currency.

2. Use the Donate Your Weight *Check*-list to track each time you perform one of the Seven Stress-Free Slimming Strategies.

3. At the end of each evening, reward yourself by putting money in your bank. Take a deep breath and acknowledge your success.

4. At the end of each week, take cash out of your can and replace small coins and bills with higher denomination bills. This serves two purposes: 1) it gives you a sense of the big picture, and 2) you can re-use your coins and small bills again the following week.

5. Repeat the process until you have reached your goal.

As you begin to experience the benefits of a trimmer, healthier, energetic body, these feelings will become your reward. Eventually you will want to follow the Strategies simply because they feel good and natural. In the process of reaching your goal you will learn to enjoy the benefits of your new behaviors and feel a sense of accomplishment each time you achieve them. Therefore, it is more likely that your new behavior changes will remain a permanent part of your life.

Creating a Plan for Your Reward Bank

Eventually, your mind might lose interest in the daily reward bank. In order to keep the momentum and motivation going, you'll want to choose a few extra special rewards throughout the process that will rekindle the excitement and keep your enthusiasm alive. For example, if you are working in a group, your group might decide to cash in all money from all members each week and put the sum total in an account or to make a weekly on-line donation to CARE at www.donateyourweight.org. Collecting all money weekly will help you to keep track of your growing total which can be a form of inspiration. Read the group instructions later in this chapter, there I'll describe how to set a vision for your group. Rather than have me tell you when and how you should donate your money, I'd rather show you how to set your own vision that is meaningful and motivating for your unique group characteristics.

If you choose to work as an individual, you will want to decide on a series of intermittent rewards throughout the process or an "end result" reward. In other words, at some point you'll cash out the money in your bank to purchase something that is special and meaningful for you. There are many ways to use these rewards as yet another way to stay motivated and on track. Ultimately it will be your personality and desires that determine what type of reward plan to follow.

For example, if you are struggling in the beginning of your program or impatient with your results, you might decide to cash in your bank every week and use the money for a non-food reward. On the other hand, if you are enjoying the reward process and are more motivated by one big reward versus a series of small rewards, you might set a goal to cash in at $100 or you might decide to keep saving until you reach a pre-determined goal such as enough money for a Swedish massage or a Hawaiian vacation.

Some participants might have money struggles or impulsive behavior that makes it difficult to feel comfortable with keeping money around. Others might live in an environment where they are concerned that someone else will find the money and spend it. If you fear that you will be tempted to spend the money on something other than what you originally decided to spend it on, or if you fear the money will somehow "disappear," you might want to consider cashing in weekly and opening a special savings account where the money will be out of daily reach. You can use your savings passbook and the growing balance as motivation instead.

One of my clients decided to use decorative marbles to track her successes. She placed these marbles in a clear vase on her dining room table and assigned a monetary amount to each marble. Each week she put money into a savings account that was equivalent to the amount of money she "donated" during the week with her marbles. Another client was not able to afford any monetary reward but she wanted to benefit from the power of rewarding her behavior. She created a decorative reward poster and put it on the wall so she would see it daily. She placed colorful stickers on it for each success she achieved. This helped her to remain positive and motivated.

Some people will put pennies in the bank each day. Others will put in quarters or maybe even dollars so, the amounts collected and the way the money is spent will vary significantly. These factors are not nearly as important as the overall big picture which can be summed up in these points:

1. Rewards motivate behavior change
2. Rewards must be feasible to be effective
3. You must follow through on the goal you set for yourself in order to be eligible for the reward
4. You must choose a reward that's exciting and motivating enough for you so that you'd rather have the reward than act on the old behavior
5. You must reward yourself often enough so that you don't feel discouraged and want to give up.

As you have noticed, this book provides strategies you can use for the rest of your life. You will never have to "go off" the Donate Your Weight program because it is a comprehensive, doable set of behaviors and techniques that will continue to enhance your life even after you reach your desired shape and size. Sometimes, getting started on a life-long journey can be daunting. That's why it's recommended that you work in groups and focus on a bigger picture versus the ups and downs of day to day life. Working in a group gives you the power to achieve your goals with greater ease as you garner the support of others and utilize the power of purpose. Research shows that group support is a vital component of life-long change.

Start a Donate Your Weight Group

In a Donate Your Weight to charity group you'll combine your personal desire for weight loss and freedom from dieting with a sense of working toward a greater cause and helping those less fortunate than yourself. The benefit of this type of plan is that your focus is on a larger cause and not the day to day tedium that can sometimes be associated with making life-long change in behavior and habits. For some, our weight problem is also tied in with a micro-focus on food and our weight. We zero in on every bite we eat and every quarter pound fluctuation in our weight. We think this micro-focus will help us achieve our goals, but in truth it prevents us from attaining the very thing we want. That said, another benefit of the "Donate Your Weight to charity" philosophy, combined with the reward bank, is that we can take the micro-focus off of ourselves and instead focus on being a positive contribution in the world. For many, the joy and satisfaction that comes from selflessly helping others can be so fulfilling that addictive and compulsive behaviors begin to subside automatically. This is a strong reason why some people have experienced great success in 12-step groups, because they focus on helping others.

Many of us have become conditioned to expect instant results. When we don't get instant results, we feel like giving up. The Donate Your Weight program is designed to help you see results all along the way. With each *Check* on your *Check*-list and each reward in your bank you are in the process of change. Focusing on a goal above and beyond your personal weight loss helps you to stick to the program and allows the results to happen naturally and without judgment or unrealistic, impatient expectations.

There are many types of groups you can form. In this section, I will describe four different types of groups. Then, at the end of the book I will provide you with a sample group format to help you get started. You can start a group that fits into one of the following categories or design your own group based on your individual circumstances.

- Peer Support Group
- Professional-Lead Support Group
- Organizational Group
- e-Group

Peer Support Group

Probably the biggest obstacle to overcome in starting your group is to let go of any ideas like, "I don't know anyone who'd want to be in the group." I often hear this claim from class, group and workshop participants. Yet the people who make the claim are themselves very interested in the group. The truth is, there are hundreds, even thousands, maybe millions of people who are craving a group like this. They are desperately searching for this. Trust me. As you begin to think of peers to join you, here are some avenues you might want to explore:

- Old diet buddies
- People you met at your last diet program
- People you met at Anonymous meetings
- People you went to/go to school with
- Co-workers
- People you met at the gym
- Members of an association or club you currently belong to
- Master Mind partners

Once you have group members, you will want to collaborate with each other regarding the frequency, location and length of your meetings. In general, weekly meetings of 1-1 ½ hours in length should be fine. The location of your group is based on convenience and group needs. You can meet in a living room, coffee shop, café or office based on what works best for all involved. You may have to play around with several locations to find one that fits your group. Try to avoid choosing a place with distractions such as the phone, kids or customers. Set this time aside for you and your goals only. This is a positive, supportive time where you allow your dreams to grow. A Donate Your Weight support group format is available in Appendix 1.

Professional-Lead Support Group

A professional-lead support group can be led by a therapist, doctor, coach, hypnotherapist, or other helping professional who has clients that desire freedom from dieting and a long-term weight loss solution. This group can operate similar to a peer group except there are added benefits to having a professional lead the group.

1. A professional can help group members stay on track and insure that the meeting sessions don't go off-topic.
2. A professional can encourage members to keep their focus on success and the process of change rather than setbacks or slow-progress.
3. A professional can address some of the deeper emotional issues that can be related to weight struggles such as childhood sexual abuse, sexual assault, anger, depression, poor self-esteem and body image issues.

4.   A professional can advise individualized interventions that will complement the Donate Your Weight program and help the client work on a more holistic level.

5.   A professional can end the group sessions with a customized visualization or hypnosis session versus using a prerecorded CD.

Professionals can utilize the format within this book and also link to the Donate Your Weight affiliate program as a way to purchase support materials at a discounted rate. See www.donateyourweight.com/affiliates for details.

Organizational Group

If you own or manage a gym, corporation, women's organization, church, or other large group, you can implement the Donate Your Weight fundraising campaign as a motivational, team building and wellness activity. Benefits of launching a Donate Your Weight campaign include:

1.   It's a wonderful opportunity to make a difference in your community and the world at large.

2.   It offers a model to help people change negative habits in a positive way.

3.   You can use the campaign to gain positive press for your organization and the charity you support.

Imagine a campaign where you help a large group of people to make positive changes in their lives while at the same time, you support a worthy cause. It doesn't get much better than that. You can use the group format in the back of the book to run structured meetings or you can encourage members to do the individual program at home, then bring their donation each week to be added to the organization total. For example, you can say, "ABC Salon is going to participate in the Donate Your Weight fundraiser from January to March. We plan to raise $10,000 for CARE and get off diets for good!" Then you can provide interested people with information on how to get started. As a group you can motivate each other to reach personal and organizational goals. (For support and creative ideas, and promotional materials or to book a speaker to come to your organization, please contact Donate Your Weight at info@ donateyourweight.com or (866)DON8-UW8.)

e-Group

If your schedule or geographical location makes it difficult for you to form a live, face-to-face group meeting, you can form or join an on-line group. Go to www.donateyourweight.com/bbs and join the message boards. Look for the forum called "Donate Your Weight support group" and post your desire to form a support group and connect with others who desire life-long freedom from the oppression of diets.

Regardless of the type of group you form, your Donate Your Weight group has a common bond because it is comprised of people who are committed to staying slim without dieting. Donate Your Weight group members are also committed to striving for a larger, more meaningful goal of helping those in need. Group support can be invaluable to long-term success. Let's face it, try as you may to say bye-bye to dieting, you will be bombarded daily with diet ads, diet claims, diet miracles, and office chit-chat regarding diets. You can't escape it completely. Working with a group gives you a feeling of assurance that you're not alone, you're not crazy, and you can do it. A positive support group can help you keep track of, and remember, your weekly progress. It can give you a boost when you feel like giving up.

A Donate Your Weight support group keeps the focus on success, positive changes made, and future desires. Save lengthy discussions about challenges or frustrations for conversations between group time with group members and other members of your broader life support system. During Donate Your Weight group time, keep your focus on what you want to grow in your life. If you keep your focus on positive changes, you'll have even more positive changes.

Points to Consider Before Starting Your Group

Before getting started, there are a couple of points to consider. Remember, a key factor in motivation and success is to know what you want to accomplish before you get started. Wayne Dyer states it this way: "Begin with the end in mind." Many self-help and hypnosis programs talk about focusing on the end result. In other words, for your group to be successful and cohesive, it will help to establish a long-term group goal and/or vision.

If you're doing the Donate Your Weight program as a group or organization, choose a cause that you are very passionate about. Donate Your Weight has chosen to affiliate with CARE because they dedicate their services to women and children and they literally feed the starving children in Africa. We love the idea of breaking old, defeating habits based on silly concepts like "finish everything on your plate, there are children starving in Africa." With Donate Your Weight and CARE you can do Strategy #2, "Leave some food on your plate" and literally help the children starving in Africa at the same time.

Once you have decided who to donate money to and how, you'll want to decide on a group goal or a group vision. Work as a team to formulate a group vision statement and read it at the beginning of each meeting to help you remember the big picture. My favorite equation for developing a vision comes from an eBook titled *Clarifying the Goal* by Ahman. His formula is $V=P+G+M$ where:

V=Vision—Vision is based on the following components (P, G and M.) It is not necessarily something you can actually see or touch but something you aspire to create or accomplish.

P=Purpose—What is the purpose for your goals? What is the "big picture?"

G=Goal—What do you specifically hope to accomplish and how?

M=Motive—What is the inner drive? What are you passionate about? Is it freedom from diets or is it feeding starving children in Africa? Is it doing something meaningful for the world or is it staying healthy so you can be there for your family?

Feel free to use this format or any other format that is familiar or useful to you. The overall purpose of creating a vision is to help motivate your activities, help you stay on track and help you remember why you're doing what you're doing.

Once you have a clear sense of your vision you can create a reward bank that will become a tool for focusing on your vision. Why not decorate your can with pictures and words that symbolize the vision and the positive things you will do with the money you collect? This will provide one more way for you to focus on the big picture and stay motivated each day to continue striving for your goals.

Maximize Your Motivation, Commitment, and Impact with the Help of Sponsors

It's one thing to collect money within your group and between members, but imagine the impact you could have if you garnered the support of sponsors. Many of us are familiar with the process of running or walking in an organized event and raising money for charity. Why not utilize this same concept in conjunction with your Donate Your Weight program? Many people have found that when they have people sponsoring their efforts financially it causes them to feel more committed to hang in for the long haul because they don't want to disappoint their friends and family members. Imagine the excitement and sense of meaning that would build for you and your group when you can donate hundreds or thousands of dollars to charity versus the smaller amount you'd be capable of securing based on your individual efforts alone. Remember, giving helps everyone involved; the giver and the receiver. Here's a sample script of what you might write or say to get the support of your prospective sponsor:

Dear _____:

As you know, I've been off and on diets for _____ years. I'm sick of diets and the temporary results. I have learned that diets will never solve my weight problem and in fact, diets have been part of the problem. I've decided to do something totally different. It's called Donate Your Weight and it will help me learn strategies I can use for the rest of my life. I'm going to commit to this program for at least _____ months before I even consider giving up. Part of my program is to save money in a reward bank each day so I can keep track of my successes. I plan to follow the program daily and raise _____ for charity to show my commitment level. I'm asking for your support to help me stay committed. The ways you can help are to:

- *Agree to match my funds*
- *Sponsor me at $ _____ per month/pound lost*
- *Sponsor me at a dollar amount that feels right to you*

All the money goes straight to charity. You can donate on-line at www.donateyourweight.org or you can write a check to CARE. All the money will help women and children and will feed starving children in Africa.

Thanks for you support.

Donate Your Weight for the Individual

The ideal way to get the most from the Donate Your Weight program is to work in a group. However, if this is impossible for you, you can still implement the program in the following way:

1. Use the Donate Your Weight *Check*-list and follow the Stress-Free Slimming Strategies daily.
2. Put money in your reward bank each evening.
3. Decide on a personal reward and make a plan for the money you will accumulate. If you're doing this program independently, you can choose to donate the money to yourself and use it for anything from a manicure to a Caribbean Cruise. Or, you can donate to charity at www.donateyourweight.org.
4. Continue with your reward plan until you reach your goal or until all behaviors become somewhat automatic for you.
5. Join us at the Donate Your Weight message boards (www.donateyourweight.com/bbs) to check in with participants from around the world and get feedback and support.
6. Utilize the resources listed in the back of this book.

PART III

CREATING LASTING
SUCCESS

CHAPTER 6

OVERCOMING POTENTIAL ROADBLOCKS WITH HEALTHY DETOURS

Now that you've got your action plan in effect, you'll want to support yourself in sticking with it over time. Roadblocks and setbacks are a normal part of life. Planning ahead to deal with them gives you an extra edge in helping you stay on track. Some roadblocks come from other people and are seemingly "out of our control." Other roadblocks are self-created and only we can change them. With creativity and honesty we may even find that sabotage from others that seems to be out of our control is actually more in our control than we care to admit. Here are some of the most common roadblocks, along with some detours to use so that you can continue moving forward on your path to a slender, healthy body.

Detour #1: Keep at It, Because You're Worth it

Roadblock #1 is wanting to give up. The key ingredient to lasting weight release is *repetition*. The most important thing you can do is to *keep taking the action* to get the results you want and maintain them.

The techniques and ideas outlined in this book are powerful and they work. Some of them are downright simple, easy, and fun compared to the methods you've tried in the past. However, it's important to remember that persistence is the key to long-term success.

The most basic rule of success is to keep on keeping on and never give up. If you plant positive thoughts and feed your mind with positive visualizations, a positive outcome is what will grow and manifest in the garden of your mind.

Weight release and maintenance takes time and is a process. Don't give up early, or keep all your focus on the final goal. Simply take your daily steps and be patient. Luckily, you don't have to be perfect to be successful. If you skip a day (or a month) of taking the steps necessary to change, just start them up again right away and get back on track as soon as possible. Don't beat yourself up for the times you don't take the steps; rather, reward yourself aplenty when you do.

There might be times when it seems like all you ever do is work and work yet you see no results. You may think "What's the point?" Maybe you'll have times when you gain weight or you stay the same weight for a long time. This can happen, but remember, you can stop the negative spiral or break through the plateau if you believe in yourself. You can make positive change. *Don't give up.* Keep on keeping on. Be honest with yourself, reevaluate, *but don't give up on yourself!*

Think about it this way. How many years have you been:

- Struggling with your weight?
- Concerned about your weight?
- Obsessed with your weight?
- Disgusted by your weight?
- Oblivious to your weight?
- In denial about your weight?

And think of this: how many years have you focused on your flaws and fat? Have you said any of the following things to yourself or felt any of the following feelings?

- "I'm so fat."
- "I'm such a cow."
- "I look like a blimp."
- "I look disgusting."
- "I'm so pathetic."
- "I'm just worthless."
- "I hate my (butt, legs, chest, waist, skin, feet, toes, fingers, ears, nose, eyes, etc …)."

It will take time to undo the effects of years of negative, self-defeating self-talk. You can't expect to undo twenty years of damage in one week! Daily practice and focus with new self-talk will begin to make a real and noticeable difference as time goes by.

How many times have you lost weight, only to gain it back? How many diets have you quit after only a few days or weeks? Aren't you sick of that? Wouldn't you love to find your ideal weight and stay there comfortably? Well, it can happen, but it won't happen overnight. You can't undo thirty years of programming in thirty days, but you sure can make a dent. The more dedicated you are, the quicker and more substantial the rewards.

A life-long journey is something that's part of your life until you die. It's not something you try out for a few weeks and then decide not to do. It's a never-ending process that requires evaluation and changing as life moves forward. Think of the word "lifestyle" and begin to integrate positive habits into your daily routine so you just become a naturally thin person. Begin observing and analyzing all your automatic habits and gradually change old habits one by one.

Everyone is different; some of us need to revamp everything in our life and others of us only need to make slight adjustments here and there. But following the Seven Stress-Free Slimming Strategies is key to creating and establishing your new lifestyle. After a good deal of time, you may find that these positive habits become ingrained and unconscious parts of your day. But for at least the first year or two, you'll want to treat them as very conscious efforts in your endeavor to care for yourself and your body in the way you truly deserve.

When you eat, start to slowly think of foods in terms of their overall value, contribution, or impact on your body. There are no "bad" foods, but moderation and variety are important, as is a balanced diet. Fresh fruits and vegetables are extremely important for the vitamins, minerals, fiber, and antioxidants they carry. You can't get these resources more efficiently in any other form.

If you have a history of being obsessed with food or weight, you will need to learn a balance between your obsession for perfection and a realistic plan for eating all through life. Some of us set unrealistic, perfectionist standards for eating that are doomed to fail. This sets up a spiral of negativity and leaves us feeling "not good enough." Perfectionism and the stress it causes can actually increase overeating and other self-defeating behaviors thereby causing us to stay stuck or go backwards versus moving forward. Focus on following the Seven Stress-Free Slimming Strategies, and allow yourself to eat all foods in moderation. The more you take care of yourself and your body, the more you'll start to enjoy and crave healthy, nourishing foods as the bulk of your meals. Still, you can always enjoy your old favorites in moderation from here on out, there's no need to demonize them.

Detour #2: Admit that You're Worth Taking the Time

Roadblock #2 is telling yourself you "don't have time for all of this." Many of us feel like we don't have time to eat healthily, enjoy our meals, and get exercise. It's time to take a realistic look at your schedule. Do you make time in your life to eat and prepare healthy meals? It does take time: trips to the grocery store, loading and unloading from the car, preparation time for the food (washing, chopping, cutting, seasoning, marinating), cooking time, and clean up time. If you work sixteen hours a day, you won't have adequate time to plan for your health. Reassess your schedule. What can stay, what needs to go? Are you willing to sacrifice your life for the sake of your work, or would you rather sacrifice some of your work for a better life? Your health is ultimately your choice, and you deserve to choose the very best for your health and well-being.

- You can follow this program very well in roughly one hour a day, which includes a balance of physical activity, conscious eating, feeding the mind, and pampering yourself every single day. If you think that's far too much time to take out of your busy schedule, consider the following points:
- Aren't you worth one hour a day of your time?
- Who gets the remaining twenty-three hours of your day?
- How many minutes, hours, days, and years have you wasted being consumed with food and weight?
- Are you ready to be free from self-hatred and obsession regarding your weight and eating?
- Wouldn't it be nice to focus on peaceful, loving, empowering thoughts versus negative, draining, and defeating thoughts?
- Think how much time you'll uncover when you feel energized, positive, and confident!

Here are some timesaving tips:
1. Say your affirmations out loud in the shower as you wait for the hair conditioner to go to work, or laminate them at your local photocopy shop and put them in your shower so you can read them aloud as you bathe.
2. Listen to your recorded affirmations while you exercise, do chores, drive, or shop.
3. Say your affirmations and/or do seated exercises at your desk chair as you wait for a print job, the computer to boot, a file to download or any other "dead" time that's an automatic part of our automated lives.

4.   Say affirmations on the commode. My favorites are "I have a very fast metabolism," and "My body processes everything I eat rapidly and efficiently." You can even say "I'm flushing the fat away," as you activate the flushing lever on your toilet.

5.   Wake up early and write in your affirmation journal first thing. When you start your day on a positive, nurturing note, it's amazing how much smoother the rest of your day goes.

Detour #3: Accept Your Body as It Is Now and Be Patient with the Process

Roadblock #3 is comparing yourself harshly to others. Your size, shape, weight, and height are individual aspects of who you are as much as your hair color, eye color, and skin color are. You cannot, and will not, look exactly like anyone else unless you are an identical twin. Continually dreaming, wishing, hoping, and working to look like someone else is self-defeating, especially if that "someone else" is a model or actress. Remember, usually when we see models and actresses they are made up, well-lit, computer-enhanced, and color-corrected images. They look pretty different in real life, which is not to say they aren't also beautiful individuals, simply that they are equally as beautiful and unique as you are.

The more you take good care of your body, the more you'll start to love it. Whenever you start to feel a comparison to someone else coming on, replace it with a statement like, "My body is uniquely beautiful," "I have the right to determine what is attractive by my own standards" or "I appreciate the way I look like no one else in the world." Feed your mind with these positive thoughts, and eventually you'll come to believe their inherent truth.

Remember, the Donate Your Weight plan is a journey, not a destination. You are constantly in the process of change. If you enjoy the process and notice the successes you achieve long the way, you'll probably experience periods of inner peace and happiness. If you are impatient with the process or yourself, or if you refuse to acknowledge any of the small successes and milestones along the way, you'll likely be agitated, annoyed, and discontent. These feelings create stress and can lead to overeating or falling off of your plan. Since your body is what it is right now and since hating it or disapproving of it won't change it, it's best to just accept it as it is while also taking positive steps to change it—if that's what is healthy and desirable for you.

Detour #4: Praise Yourself for Every Positive Step You Take

Roadblock #4 is self-criticism and never feeling "good enough." During the process of becoming a naturally thin person, you are likely to have bad days—maybe even bad weeks. The old diet/perfectionist mentality may creep back up, and you may find yourself starting to "beat yourself up" and focus on all you didn't do and how "bad" you've been. You might even feel like a loser or failure or have fluctuations in your weight. If this happens, just say, "It's okay," and continue to do the best you can anyway. Don't give up and don't judge yourself. None of us is perfect, so we can just give up on that now. We never will be perfect, whatever that even means.

Remember, what you focus on gets stronger. Focus on every success you have, regardless of how small and insignificant it may seem. At the end of each day, "Donate Your Weight" for every single success you have, and each day when you pamper yourself, remind yourself that you're doing a great job. If you struggle with remembering all that you've done well, keep your Success *Check-*list handy so you'll have a visual reminder of all you've done right. You can also get a success journal and log every positive step you take. Give yourself credit for all the times you choose a new way of doing things and every time you do the steps outlined in the book. Forgive yourself for all times you fall short. Focus your energy on where you want to go and eventually you will get there.

Detour #5: Magnify Your Successes and Your Positive Traits

Roadblock #5 is magnifying your perceived flaws. We all have different shapes. Top heavy, bottom heavy, curvy, flat, thick thighs, short waists, and on and on. You can find creative ways to accentuate or optimize your shape but in general, you aren't likely to permanently change your body's natural shape. So it's important to accept the dimensions of your body now and find a way to feel good about them. Sometimes what we perceive as ugly or a flaw can be seen as a beauty mark or unique characteristic. Think of Barbara Streisand's nose or the gap between Lauren Hutton and Madonna's front teeth. How about Jennifer Lopez and her infamous behind, or the mole on Cindy Crawford or Marilyn Monroe's face? Can you find a way to love your "flaw?" Act "as if" it's your unique, fabulous, and wonderful mark in society. Embrace it.

On the flipside, why not magnetize your strengths and abilities. Take time to think daily about your successes and the things you handled positively during the day. Keep a running list of things you're grateful for and things you like about yourself. Create a scrapbook filled with pleasant memories and successful events on each page. Review these items regularly and give all your attention to these positive aspects until they become your primary focus. Take the emphasis away from your negative thoughts about yourself and put it on positive thoughts instead.

Detour #6: Release Worry and Take Action to Prevent Weight Gain

Roadblock #6 is fears of eventual weight gain. Many of the steps outlined in this book ask you to work toward a new mindset regarding food and your body. Techniques such as affirmations and visualization are used to strengthen your belief system so you can get in touch with your inner strength and your body's ability to guide you to right choices. In a sense, the affirmations and visualizations help you to build faith, and fear is the antithesis of faith. Therefore, each time you start to feel afraid about your weight, it's important to make a conscious effort to turn it around and remind yourself of all of your positive efforts and your faith in yourself and the process. Remember, what you focus on tends to grow, so focus on the positive changes you've made.

You can also focus on the facts: you would need to eat 3,500 extra calories above what your body burns in a day in order to gain one pound. So when you have a piece of cake, remind yourself that this in itself isn't going to "pack on the pounds." Even if you do eat enough to gain a pound, taking action will serve you much better in the long run than worrying. So each time you start feeling especially afraid of backsliding, increase your affirmation and self-hypnosis time, as well as your pamper time, because for something to really work as a lifestyle, it has to feel genuinely pleasurable and rewarding.

Detour #7: Release Unrealistic Expectations and Embrace Yourself

Roadblock #7 is getting stuck in unrealistic expectations. Unrealistic expectations lead to discouragement, failure, defeat, dissatisfaction, low self-esteem, and more undesirable results. Nothing positive *ever* comes out of unrealistic expectations, no matter how much you hope they will "motivate" you. In this section, we'll review some common types of unrealistic expectations and ways you can deal with them.

Releasing Unrealistic Expectations Regarding Size and Weight

Some of us decide on a size/weight goal based on past experience. We decide we want to weigh the same as we did twenty years ago, because that's when we really felt thin. Can you truly expect to attain and maintain a weight from your youth based on your current lifestyle? Can you be happy and sane doing so? One way to determine a realistic weight is to look at the BMI (Body Mass Index) chart. My favorite tool is available at the National Heart Lung and Blood Institute website[6] it's an electronic calculator that automatically computes your BMI after you enter your height and weight. You can also type "Body Mass Index Chart" into any search engine and find a variety of other charts and formulas to calculate your BMI. The BMI chart helps you to find the weight that's right for you and your health. It's not based on current fashion trends.

As far as clothing size is concerned, let's remember that this number is almost meaningless. We can go to three stores and be a different size at each one. The number on the tag says nothing about the health of your body. Some of us give the tag on our clothes too much power and even limit ourselves to wearing clothes from particular outlets, designers, or manufacturers because we like the size we "get to be" when we wear them. But sizes are completely arbitrary: as a teen, I wore between a size 9 and 11, but now, as an adult I weigh more but wear a 6 or 8 most of the time. How is a system like that worth pinning all our self-esteem on?

A more accurate way to measure your body is a good, old-fashioned measuring tape. However, refrain from any temptation to measure yourself more often than monthly. Once you get to a healthy weight, you can determine if your weight/fat ratio is comfortable for you by doing a fat analysis. You may decide to engage in specific exercises that will tone your body and decrease your size. Once you find a comfortable size, let your clothing be your guide. If your clothes get tight, pay attention. Evaluate. Have you been eating more than usual or are you just temporarily bloated? If your clothes are too tight for several days, it's time to take steps that lead to a decrease in size, such as renewing your dedication to the Seven Stress-Free Slimming Strategies.

Releasing Unrealistic Expectations Regarding Weight-Release Results

Healthy weight release is ½ to 2 pounds a week. Anything faster than this and you may be jeopardizing your health. Many times we are disappointed if our weight release isn't rapid or drastic. It's important to be aware of these feelings and to be realistic with your rate of weight loss. A more accurate way to assess your progress is to monitor your activity. If you're taking the right

---

6   http://www.nhlbisupport.com/bmi/bmicalc.htm

steps consistently, the results should come. Using the scale as the gauge of your progress is frustrating and self-defeating. It's almost impossible not to experience a slight feeling of stress when the scale shows that you've maintained or gained. Stressing out over a slight gain can be self-defeating, since weight gain and stress are related. The best thing to do is repeat affirmations to yourself, stay on track, and expect the gain to be a temporary fluke. The more power and energy you give it, the more likely you are to make it come true.

Releasing Unrealistic Expectations of Our Body as We Age

It's true that metabolism does slow down with age, though partially this has to do with your muscle mass. You lose muscle mass with age and since muscle helps burn fat, you lose some of your fat-burning capacity. However, if you choose an exercise plan that includes strength training or muscle building, the effects of age are decreased (and some even claim it can be reversed). Of course, the other benefits include greater mobility, physical strength, flexibility, stamina and self-esteem. Exercise can also lead to a decrease in blood pressure, cholesterol levels, anxiety and depression. By keeping your muscles strong and flexible, you help avoid problems in late life, such as difficulties getting up, laying down, sitting, and getting from place to place.

Chances are, if you are over forty you will not return to the weight you were in high school and look good doing it. Our bodies often shift how weight is distributed as we age. A size or weight that looked great when we were sixteen may make us look bony and gaunt in our forties and beyond, especially in our faces. Be realistic with yourself and choose a weight/size that looks good on your body today. Avoid trying to reach a standard from the past that doesn't fit you today. Take an accurate assessment of your current situation and plan ahead so you can work within your needs. Honesty and flexibility are important keys to success in long-term weight maintenance.

Releasing Unrealistic Expectations Regarding How to Eat

Some dieters get trapped into thinking that the diet is the "right" way to eat and all other ways are "wrong." What they don't see is that any new food plan is just another jail in disguise, another temporary and frustrating attempt to be perfect (which is impossible). Here is a guarantee: if you expect yourself to be perfect, you will live your life in constant disappointment, which, ironically, often leads to the very self-defeating behaviors you're trying to control. If you want to find a way to be at peace with your body and food, you will need to find a balanced plan that is truly workable for you and flexible enough for life's unexpected dilemmas and pleasant surprises.

Releasing Unrealistic Expectations Regarding How to Look

Some of us are filled to the brim with unrealistic ideals regarding how we should look. Our minds are filled with images from magazines and TV, and sometimes we may compare ourselves unfavorably to family members or friends. We may want perfectly flat stomachs and cellulite-free bottoms. We may want to eliminate all fat rolls and abolish all signs of imperfection. Many times, the images we hold in our minds are like a carrot dangled in front of a horse—always just out of reach. In order to have sanity in our lives, we need to be realistic and we need to learn to love and embrace those "flaws"—cellulite, stretch marks and pockets of fat are a fact of life for most women, even thin women!

We need to take an honest assessment of ourselves, our age, our lifestyle, and our level of commitment so we can establish a realistic goal. If you are willing and capable to do hard exercise daily or most days (though this is something you'll need to slowly work up to, or else you may get injured or discouraged), you can have higher expectations. But if you're a full-time parent, full-time employee, full-time student, or a combination of two or more of those things, you can't realistically expect to have time for a perfectly balanced diet and a rigid exercise program. However, you *can* attain a slender, attractive, and healthy weight, and you can maintain it. Finding realistic goals and maintaining them are keys to success and happiness on this journey.

Detour # 8: Appreciate Your Body from the Inside Out

Roadblock #8 is hating your body. Many of us began dieting at a fairly young age because we were unhappy with our bodies, and some of us can't even remember a time in our lives when we were happy with our bodies. I know a woman who was called "fatty" by the neighborhood bullies when she was seven, and for forty-five years she's heard their cruel words over and over again in her head. She repeated these words to herself probably thousands of times. She felt like a "fatty", even when she lost 70 pounds and became very slim and trim. One day, she realized how much power she gave these neighborhood kids over all the years. She decided to take back her power and refused to be held hostage to this childhood incident.

Diet mentality has reduced our thoughts about ourselves to a list of complaints about our butt, thighs, stomach and arms. In the meantime, we've completely ignored the rest of our body and we often forget all the things we have to be grateful for. Try writing a gratitude list for your body. Think about your lungs (which are helping you breathe right now), your heart (which is pumping your blood through your body this very second), your eyes (which are allowing you to read this book so you can get the help you need), and your ears, nose, mouth, fingers, toes, eyelashes, and all of the thousands of body parts that are working together in harmony to make it possible for you to be alive each day. How cruel of us to hate our body ... after all it's done for us!

Weight loss programs are primarily focused on the parts of your body you can see in a mirror. However, your body is much more than just the external excess fat you're focusing on. Your body has been carrying you around wherever you want to go, helping you see, smell, and hear some amazing things and allowing you to bend, move, reach, walk, and talk. Isn't it time to say "thank you" to your cells, your organs, your limbs, your brain, and all parts of your amazing body? Your body is an intricate, living organism that works for you twenty-four hours a day, seven days a week, without fail. It deserves your gratitude and your care.

Go to a bookstore and buy a big huge body atlas with full-color pictures. Go ahead and purchase the large book designed for children and study the pages with a sense of awe. You don't have to get a professional manual that requires you to be a doctor to understand it. Just look at the illustrations and read the simple explanations to get a glimpse of what a miracle your body truly is. Your body is not disgusting, it's your home. Get to know it, and marvel at how your muscles, veins, arteries, bones, organs, and glands all work in harmony to keep you alive. The human body is much smarter than the newest technological gadget: how many computers do you know of that can cure themselves of a virus? Next time you cut yourself or get a bruise, notice how your body goes to work immediately to heal your skin.

Let's face it, most of us are guilty of taking our body for granted. All this amazing stuff happens in our bodies effortlessly and daily for many, many years, and most of us are completely oblivious and ungrateful. It's time to give the body the respect it deserves. Let's stop overstuffing or starving it. Let's stop treating it so neglectfully that we'd be thrown in jail for severe abuse and neglect if we were behaving this way toward another person.

Here are a few other reasons to appreciate your body: You couldn't go on vacations if it wasn't for your body. You would never be able to watch a movie, read a book, or take a walk if it wasn't for your body. You'd never hear music if it wasn't for your body. So go get that body atlas and look at it page by page. Look at it until any feelings of disgust are replaced with complete awe and gratitude. Really thank your body for being there for you. The better you treat it, the better it will treat you.

Detour #9: Put the Scale in Perspective

Roadblock #9 is letting the scale determine your self-esteem. One of the ways we can sabotage our success and make ourselves miserable is to weigh ourselves daily and allow our moods to be impacted by the number we see. There are numerous reasons why the scale is not an accurate measure of your body, especially on a day-to-day basis. In fact, if you're addicted to the scale, I have an exercise for you in the spirit of paradoxical intention (prescribing the symptom): Weigh yourself every day, several times a day, for a full week. Try to eat a normal diet and normal food intake (although, chances are you might do some "scale-related" eating, another reason why daily weigh-ins are counterproductive). Nonetheless, weigh yourself as soon as you wake up then again midday, then again in the evening. Keep a running diary. Write it down so you can see any patterns. Do this for one week. Write it all down then weigh yourself again the next morning. Notice how you mysteriously "lose weight in your sleep." (Hmmmm, how does that happen?) What you will probably find after doing this exercise is that the scale makes no sense. You may find yourself losing and gaining as much as 5 pounds within one day. The fluctuations you see are primarily water changes. As soon as you use the bathroom or sweat or just evaporate (yes, we lose water even in our normal day-to-day operations), the scale's reading will change. This change has nothing whatsoever to do with your body shape, size, or fat content. A pound of feathers and a pound of lead will weigh the same yet look drastically different.

Think of your body as a kitchen scrub sponge that stays the same size whether wet or dry. Imagine a brand new, soft sponge right out of the package. It is light and airy. Now, fill it with water and pick it up. It's still the same size but now it's heavier. As soon as you wring it out, it will get lighter again. Your body is constantly absorbing and releasing water throughout the day but that has nothing to do with getting fat.

Another important note: your digestive tract is 30 feet long from beginning to end. That's about the length of a train car, though most of your digestive tract is compacted and twisted into a space that's 6 by 10 inches. When you eat food, it takes at least three to ten hours for it to make its trek from the beginning of your digestive tract to the end. During that time, you might weigh more but you didn't gain weight. Of course a variety of factors will impact your rate of digestion. Higher fiber foods tend to digest quicker. Meat takes the longest, especially red meat. Fruits and vegetables tend to digest quickly. Exercise and water intake can also impact your digestive rate.

That pound or two you gain throughout the day is not from the food you eat and it's not fat. Remember, it requires 3,500 calories over and above what you need to maintain your weight in order for you to gain even one pound. A small cookie has about 50 calories, so you'd have to eat seventy cookies over and above all the calories you needed to fuel your body for the day in order for you to be at potential risk for gaining the dreaded one pound. A scoop of ice cream has about 150 to 200 calories, so you'd have to eat eighteen to twenty-four servings to gain a pound (a half gallon of ice cream contains sixteen servings). So, next time you see a gain on the scale, use logic instead of emotionalism to explain the change. Take the power away from the scale. Even better, stop using the scale all together. There are other, more accurate ways to gauge your progress such as your clothing size. If you get too upset with what you see on the scale, it could actually lead to overeating, which is counterproductive to your goal.

On a mind/body communication level, each trip to the scale is equal to "checking." It's as if you're saying to yourself, "I don't believe I'm making any positive changes, so I'd better check." Each time you "check" you are negating all other forms of change and giving all the power to the scale. This lack of trust will be counterproductive to your long-term goals. Remember, the scale cannot measure your improved self-esteem, your ability to control food choices, your behavior changes, or the changes in the composition or shape of your body. All a scale can measure is the pull of gravity on mass. And that's no way to measure your worth.

Detour #10: Embrace Your Favorite Foods and Beverages

Roadblock #10 is slipping back into diet mentality and labeling some foods as "bad." Your favorite foods and beverages must be a part of your ongoing menu. Whether it's pizza, doughnuts, peanuts, or alcohol, you need to find a moderate, acceptable way to enjoy your favorite foods and beverages on a fairly regular basis. Remember, you are learning to live without restrictive dieting. You can technically have these foods anytime you want. So you can choose when and how much, and you don't have to "eat it all right now." You can even choose to take a few bites just for the taste. Diet mentality leads you to think you are "bad" when you eat sweets and therefore "might as well eat it all, since I failed anyway." However, when you take your judgments off of it, you can choose to eat the food or not. It's not bad, you're not bad, you simply made a food choice. It may not have been the healthiest choice possible, but then we don't always have to make the healthiest choice possible in every moment. That would make us superhuman saints. So remember, eating your favorite food from time to time doesn't make you a bad person and it doesn't mean you're going to die. As you strive to create balance and health in your life, you will begin automatically gravitating to healthier choices.

Detour #11: Take Complete Responsibility for Your Actions and Outcomes

Roadblock #11 is holding on to weight because of fear or old ideas. Remember, thoughts are powerful. If your thoughts and memories are focused on the past, you miss out on the freedom that's available in the present moment. You have what it takes to reach your weight-reduction goals. Really you do. But if your mind or body is telling you "I'm not ready" or "this will never work," you might be experiencing backlash from emotional baggage and negative beliefs about your ability to be slender and healthy. This will need to be addressed if you wish to reach your goal and tackle this problem for good. You have to learn to confront the attitudes, beliefs, behaviors, and fears related to being thin and staying thin.

Living with unresolved emotional issues and a weight problem takes time and energy. If you could release your painful feelings and negative beliefs, establish ongoing healthy habits, and get to a healthy weight, what will you do with all the free time that this would create (given that you no longer have to spend all day beating yourself up)? How will you channel all the energy you've been using to "fight" your weight problem all these years? How will you handle not being able to obsess on food and your body? What will it be like to not have to struggle with your weight? What will it mean if you actually liked and accepted yourself as you are—imperfections and all?

For some of us, when we really slow down and think about it, we have to admit it's scary as all heck to just let our minds be quiet and live in the truth of every moment. However, the current moment is where all your power resides. Dwelling on the past will rob you of the energy you have today. When old emotions from the past are deeply rooted, some find it beneficial to seek professional help. If you choose to seek professional help, be sure to tell the person you're working with all about this book and the goals you're trying to reach. If the professional tries to talk you out of your goal, or insists that you delve into your pain and that this is the "only" answer, it might be a sign that you are not a good match for this particular professional. There are volumes of research and thousands of professionals who know that focusing on problems makes the problems grow larger and more overwhelming. My favorite professionals practice therapy techniques such as:

Somatic Experiencing

Deep Emotional Release Body Work
Art Therapy
Feminist Therapy
Hypnosis
EMDR (Eye Movement Desensitization Reprocessing)
EFT (Emotional Freedom Technique)

These techniques employ a mind/body philosophy and also help you make changes at a deep, subconscious level. For more information, see the resources page in the back of this book.

Detour #12: Use Your Thoughts and Feelings as a Guide

Roadblock #12 is denying or being afraid to notice undesirable feelings. As you journey on the road to self-change you might have setbacks. You might not always be perfect. No worries. It's better to be aware of the changes you need to make than to fool yourself into thinking everything is okay when it isn't. You are a multi-faceted person with two parts of your brain often in conflict. The "old, mammalian" brain wants instant gratification, the "new, neo-cortex" wants things like peace, harmony, freedom and happiness. The concerns of all the parts of your personality need to be addressed one at a time and taken seriously, because trust me, if you try to ignore any part of you, it will continue to make things difficult for you until it's heard and taken seriously. To help facilitate this process, try the following "root down" exercise, which involves a journal and a little mental clearing. Label one column "Affirmation/Goal," in it write out your goal in the form of an affirmation (such as "I am releasing weight"). Label column two "Response," and write out any mental or physical responses you have to the statement in column one. If you are unaware of any immediate reactions, close your eyes, take a deep breath, and continue to slowly repeat the sentence from column one to yourself and write down any responses you have. Then go back to column one and write an affirmation/goal in response to the fears or misgivings of the statement in the second column. Keep going back and forth until you no longer have any negative responses to the initial statement in column one.

Here's an example:

Affirmation/Goal	Response
"I want to lose weight."	That means no more mocha's every morning. I feel deprived.
I look forward to the health, energy, and vitality I'll feel when I'm toned and thin.	Yeah, but it's so much work.
I am developing the habits of a naturally thin person. It's easy for me to stay slim.	Wow, that would be cool! But is it possible?
It is possible to be a naturally thin person if I am willing to change my attitudes and behaviors. It's possible to eat foods I like from time to time and still stay slim.	I think maybe it is. I'm willing to give it a try now. I can honestly say, "I want to lose weight."

Basically, the "root down" exercise helps you identify your resistances to change and allows you to address them directly rather than being tricked or persuaded into giving up. It's also a way for you to assure that unsure part of yourself that this change will be pleasurable and good for you.

Detour #13: Trust Your Ability to Make Wise Choices

Roadblock #13 is self-doubt or making someone else's opinion more important than your own. We live in a world of diet commercials, diet food, diet drinks and corporate diet centers. The diet industry brings in 55 billion dollars a year by selling you on the idea that diets will solve your weight problem. The diet industry uses powerful media advertising to make weight loss claims and show off its success stories. Millions of people are on some form of a diet at any given time. Then there's you. The brave soul who decided to buck the system; the wise soul who refuses to be swept away by another diet plan only to be spit out later with all your weight back and a few mental and emotional bruises to boot.

The diet industry is powerful, and so are you. There might be times however, when you feel like giving up. You might just decide you were crazy to start this program and you "should" just go back to diets like "everyone else." It's important to discuss your feelings of self-doubt with your Donate Your Weight support group. You are not crazy for trying the Donate Your Weight plan. What is crazy is to do something over and over again and expect different results. Most likely you have tried diets over and over again and most likely you always gained the weight back plus more as soon as you went off the diet. If you take a good look around you, most likely you will find that these results are typical. Diets are almost always temporary. You have to do something different if you want different results. See figure 6.1 for the typical diet results. Does it look familiar?

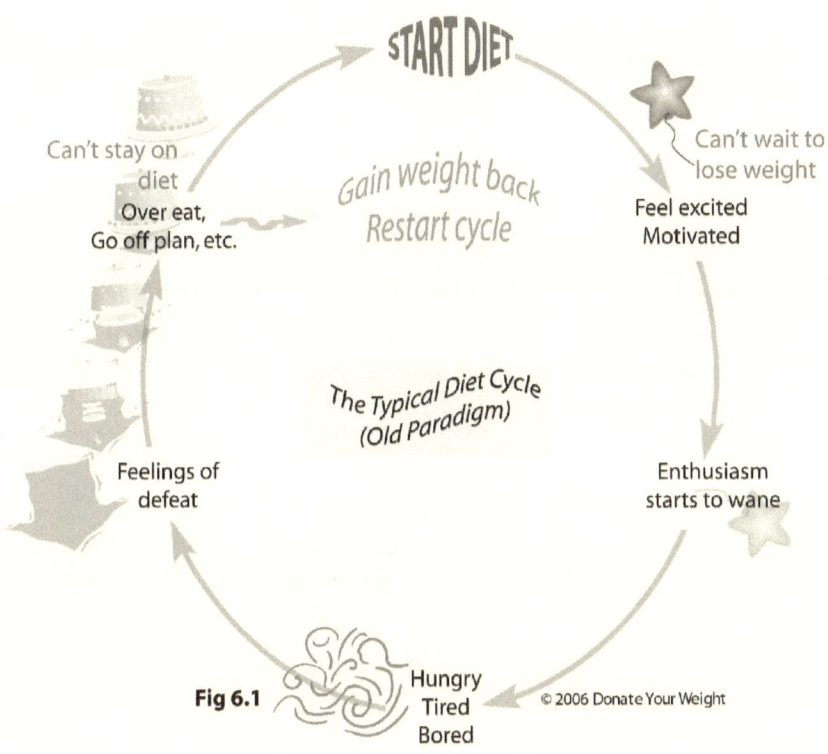

Fig 6.1

© 2006 Donate Your Weight

When you stick with the Donate Your Weight plan, you can create a new cycle that looks something like this:

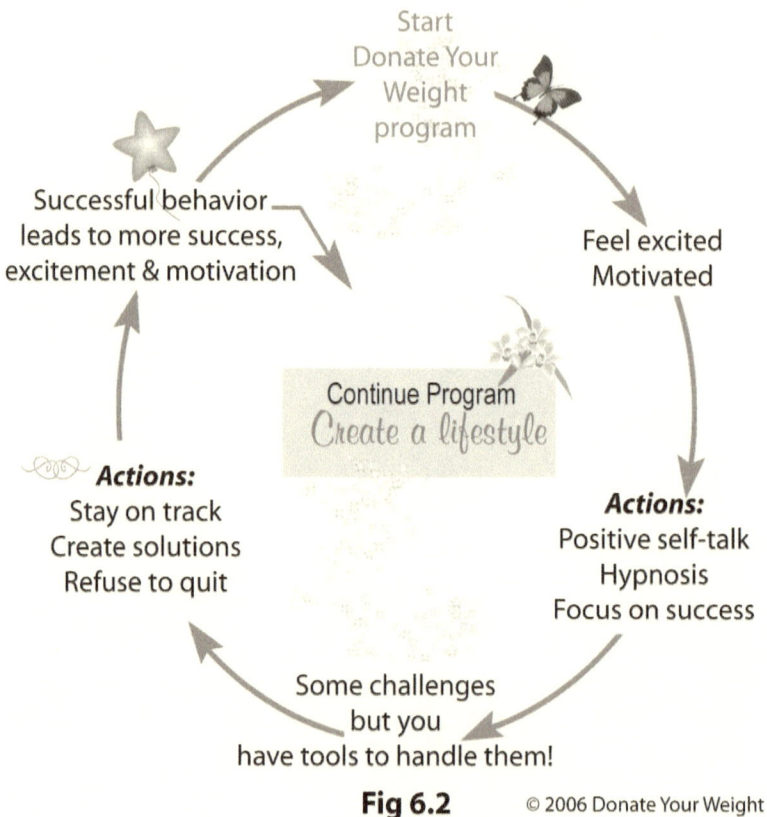

Start
Donate Your
Weight
program

Feel excited
Motivated

Successful behavior
leads to more success,
excitement & motivation

Continue Program
Create a lifestyle

Actions:
Stay on track
Create solutions
Refuse to quit

Actions:
Positive self-talk
Hypnosis
Focus on success

Some challenges
but you
have tools to handle them!

Fig 6.2   © 2006 Donate Your Weight

In Conclusion

So now you've got a set of tools, techniques, resources and ideas that can help you live a freer, more enjoyable life in relation to food and your weight. If there were one necessary ingredient that's guaranteed to make it all work it would have to be *persistence*. Keep up your Seven Stress-Free Slimming Strategies, continue to Donate Your Weight, focus on the process rather than the end result, and praise yourself for every positive step you take. Garner the support of others by starting a support group or participate in a fundraising campaign. Have fun. Don't give up. Gradually you will see your life, your attitude, and your body change in very positive ways.

An important key to persistence is to continually remind yourself of your goals and the benefits of achieving them. The following list can also help to remind you why you've chosen Donate Your Weight over dieting and why you can be proud of your decision.

Donate Your Weight	Diets
Gets easier and more enjoyable the longer you do it	Gets harder and less enjoyable the longer you do it
Results are lasting because you have created a way of life	Results are temporary. You did what someone told you to do but its not something you can do for the rest of your life
Enjoyable and fun most of the time	Stressful and boring most of the time
Feel normal because you can eat what others are eating	Feel isolated because you're on a diet and no one else around you is
Strategies can be used for life	Stick to the plan temporarily, then.... who knows?
Strategies can be used to make changes in other areas of life as well	It's all about food and weight
Focus is on daily rewards, daily progress	Focus is on weight
Focus is on establishing life-long habits	Focus is on following the plan perfectly

By making a choice to stop dieting, you have made a choice to succeed. According to a 2007 report out of UCLA which was published in *American Psychologist*, "Dieting Does Not Work,"[7] Traci Mann, UCLA associate professor of psychology and lead author of the study wrote, "We found that the majority of people regained all the weight, plus more. Sustained weight loss was found only in a small minority of participants, while complete weight regain was found in the majority." After conducting "the most comprehensive and rigorous analysis of diet studies, analyzing 31 long-term studies," Mann and her co-authors concluded that "most [people] would have been better off not going on the diet at all. Their weight would be pretty much the same, and their bodies would not suffer the wear and tear from losing weight and gaining it all back." Of course there's also the emotional and mental wear and tear of feeling like a hopeless failure. By making the decision to chart a new path, you won't have to experience the emotional, mental and physical wear and tear of dieting ever

---

7   http://newsroom.ucla.edu/portal/ucla/Dieting-Does-Not-Work-UCLA-Researchers-7832.aspx?RelNum=7832

again. Instead, you will begin a journey that gets easier with time and that will result in feelings of lasting empowerment and joy. I wish you all the best on your journey, and I hope to see you on the path.

References

American Obesity Association: http://www.obesity.org/

Annesi, James, J. "Effects of a cognitive behavioral treatment package on exercise attendance and drop out in fitness center." *Journal of Sport Science*, V3. N2. (April, 2003)

Brody, Howard. *The Placebo Response*. 2000. New York: Harper Collins.

Gulb, Stephen. *The Thin Commandments Diet: The 10 No-Fail Strategies for Permanent Weight Loss*. New York: Rodale Books.

Lisa M. Groesz, Michael P. Levine & Sarah K. Murnen. "The effect of experimental presentation of thin media images on body satisfaction: A meta-analytic review." *International Journal of Eating Disorders*. V31. Issue 1. (December, 2001)

Lehrman, Fredrick. *Prosperity Consciousness*. Chicago: Nightingale Conant.

Tribole, Evelyn & Resch, Elyse 2003. *Intuitive Eating*. St. Martin's Griffin.

Partnership for Healthy Weight Maintenance: http://www.consumer.gov/weightloss/setgoals.htm

U.S. Department of Health and Human Services: www.health.gov

Watson, David L & Tharp, Roland G. 2006 *Self-Directed Behavior*, 9th Edition.

RESOURCES

Free Resources

Each of the following free resources is available at www.donateyourweight.com.

- Weekly motivational tips—tips to help you stay on track with your new non-diet lifestyle.
- Weekly motivational podcasts—audio motivation you can listen to at your computer or download to your mp3 player.
- Donate Your Weight Blog—articles and information to help you stay on track.
- Teleseminars—monthly conference calls where you can get your questions answered and learn more about Donate Your Weight.
- Message boards—Private and public forums available to get information and meet others who are interested in Donate Your Weight.

Hypnosis and affirmation CD's/Downloads

Go to www.donateyourweight.com to see an up-to-date list of hypnosis and affirmation audio products. These products will help you to successfully implement the Seven Stress-Free Slimming Strategies into your daily life.

1. *Stress-Free Slimming*—a CD that will help you learn and live the Seven Strategies with ease
2. *It's Safe To Be Thin*—a CD all about owning your personal power and releasing fears or blocks to weight loss
3. *Love Your Body, Love Yourself*—a CD all about self-love, self-nurturing and being grateful for your body now
4. *Rev Up Your Metabolism*—a CD all about making healthy choices and focusing on the mind/body connection

Therapeutic Resources

EMDR—Eye Movement Desensitization and Reprocessing. This therapeutic technique has been highly recommended for those who need help releasing the effects of a past traumatic event. Go to http://www.emdr.com/clinic.htm#search to find a professional in your area.

EFT—Emotional Freedom Technique. This technique is touted for breaking habits and changing a negative emotional state. You can download a free packet of information at their website: http://www.emofree.com/a/?2617

Psychology Today—Find a Therapist[8]. Use this online resource to search for a therapist in your area. Remember, types of therapy that can be very beneficial to you in relation to healing past trauma and emotional issues without having to delve deeply into your past for years on end include: Somatic Experiencing, Deep Emotional Release Body Work, Art Therapy, Feminist Therapy and Hypnosis. See if you can find professionals that specialize in one or more of these areas.

---

8   http://therapists.psychologytoday.com/rms/prof_search.php

RECOMMENDED READING

Ahman. 2007. *Clarifying the Goal.* (eBook) www.inspirationsministries.org.

Guiliano, Mireille. 2004. *French Women Don't Get Fat.* New York: Knopf Publishing Group.

Hay, Louise L.1984. *You Can Heal Your Life.* Carlsbad, CA: Hay House.

Hill, Napoleon 2004. *Think and Grow Rich.* Aventine Press.

McGee, Robyn 2005. *Hungry for More.* Emeryville, CA: Seal Press.

Oliver-Pyatt, Wendy 2003. *Fed Up! Free Yourself from the Diet Trap.* New York: McGraw-Hill.

Orbach, Susie 1997. *Fat is a Feminist Issue: The Anti-Diet Guide to Permanent Weight Loss.* BBS Publishing Group.

Peale, Norman Vincent 1996. *The Power of Positive Thinking.* New York: Ballantine Books.

Podjasek, Jill 1988. *10 Habits of Naturally Thin People.* New York: McGraw-Hill.

Schaefer, Jenni 2004. *Life without Ed: How One Woman Declared Independence from Her Eating Disorder and How You Can Too.* New York: McGraw-Hill.

Schwartz, Bob. 1996. *Diets Don't Work.* Houston, TX: Breakthru Publishing.

Steinem, Gloria 1992. *Revolution from Within.* Boston: Little, Brown and Company.

Tribole, Evelyn & Resch, Elyse 2003. *Intuitive Eating.* New York: St. Martin's Griffin.

Turner, Laura 2004. *Spiritual Fitness.* Victor, NY: Violet Prose Publications.

Watson, David L & Tharp, Roland G. 2006 *Self-Directed Behavior,* 9th Edition.

Gladwell, Malcom 2000. *The Tipping Point.* New York: Little, Brown and Company.

Zampelli, Sheri O. 2002. *From Sabotage to Success.* Lincoln, NE: Back in Print. com

Zampelli, Sheri O. 2006 *Start Your Own Master Mind Group: Utilize the Seven Simple Steps to Overcome Self-Sabotage* (eBook) www.donateyourweight.com.

APPENDIX I

DONATE YOUR WEIGHT SUPPORT GROUP FORMAT

Five Steps to Start the Group:

1. Choose a leader for the meeting (ideally a Donate Your Weight support group is somewhat leaderless in that all members are equal and you choose a different person to lead each week.)

2. Leader starts the meeting by reading the group vision (see Chapter 5 for details).

3. Leader instructs all group members to read the Seven Strategies aloud in unison as a way to help the group memorize the strategies and get focused. (To download a full-color list of these strategies go to http://www.donateyourweight. com/images/7strat.pdf.)

4. Leader asks one member to read the Seven Stress-Free Slimming Strategies for Groups aloud (Appendix III).

5. Leader chooses a format from below (based on group consensus) and helps the group stay on track.

Group Format Options

Option 1: Participation Style Group:

After following the above five steps, leader starts the participation portion of the meeting by sharing her/his successes for the past week including how much she/he donated to the reward bank, as well as reports or feedback regarding the Success *Check*-list and anything new or different that has happened this week in relation to following the Donate Your Weight program.

Below is a sample sharing format for the group to follow. It's only meant as a guideline to get the group started. Feel free to modify it and remember to be flexible and forgiving of yourself when sharing.

"My name is _____. This week I donated $ _____. My successes this week were that I _____. In my success notes I wrote _____. What I noticed about myself (food, my weight, my thinking, society, etc.) is that _____."

Leader continues by stating her/his donation goal for the upcoming week and any specific action goals. For example:

"This coming week my goal is to donate $ _____ (choose a number that is the same or higher than your number for this week) and I'm going to focus specifically on Strategy 6 this week and listen to a self-hypnosis CD every day."

After leader shares her/his goals, all members make an affirmative statement to the leader in unison: ***"I believe you can do whatever you want to do."***

Leader then turns the time over to another participant and each member of the group follows the sample sharing format above until everyone has had a chance to participate.

Option 2: Book Study Style Group:

Leader begins the meeting by following the Five Steps to Start the Group. Leader then chooses a chapter from the book and reads a section from one paragraph to one page in length. Usually groups who use the Book Study format will start at the beginning of the book and progress through each chapter until they get to the end. Then, depending on the group structure, they might start the book over or choose a new book from the recommended reading list. Preferably everyone has her/his own book, if not, the leader can pass her/his book around allowing everyone to take turns reading. Reading continues until the chapter is completed or time is up. Participants can then share about how the reading impacted them, how they relate to it on a personal level or how they plan to institute what they've read into their daily life. After reading, participants can follow the participation guidelines listed in Option 1 to share successes and goals with each other.

Ending the Group Session

At the conclusion of the meeting, leader closes by expressing appreciation to everyone for their participation. Depending on the composition of the group and time available you may want to also consider including the following components to your group:

1. Elect a treasurer who will collect all charitable donations each week and make a group report.

2. End the meeting with a self-hypnosis CD or guided visualization.

DONATE YOUR WEIGHT
SUCCESS *CHECK*-LIST

Available for download at: http://www.donateyourweight.com/site/success_checklist.pdf

Donate Your Weight Weekly Success *Check*-list   Name: _____

Action Items	Sample	Monday	Tuesday	Wednesday	Thursday	Friday	Saturday	Sunday
Date:	11/20/07							
Chewed slowly 🖐🖐	✔ ✔ ✔							
Paused between bites	✔ ✔ ✔							
Stopped at "satisfaction" (before "full")	✔ ✔ ✔							
Left food on plate	✔ ✔ ✔							
Waited about 3-5 hours between meals	✔ ✔ ✔							
One *Check* for each glass of water	✔ ✔ ✔ ✔ ✔ ✔							
Exercised 20 minutes or more	✔							
Said, wrote or listened to affirmations	✔							
Listened to self-hypnosis CD	✔							
Did self-pampering	✔							
Use the lines below to add your own goal								
Total daily *Checks* 🖐	25							
						Grand Total *Checks* >>>		

🖐 🖐 Count to 10 or more while chewing each bite   ⬤ Stop before feeling full - Listen for the sigh

   Put utensil or food down while chewing   🖐 Total your *Checks* each day, then tally the grand total each week

    ✔ Now, choose a monetary reward amount for each *Check* and put it in your Donate Your Weight collection jar for self-pampering or charity

Success Notes:

(Use this area to jot down awarenesses, realizations, challenges and more.
No change is too small and if you don't write it, you might forget it.)

	Sample:	
	Total *Checks*	25
	x Money Reward	0.25
	Donation Amount	6.25
	✔ My **Weekly** Totals:	
	Grand Total *Checks* >>>	
	x Money Reward	
	Donation Amount	

© 2007 Donate Your Weight.com   Download additional checklists at : http://www.donateyourweight.com/site/success_checklist.pdf

Appendix III

Seven Stress-Free Slimming Strategies for Groups

The Seven Stress-Free Slimming Strategies have been designed to help break habits and create a new life free from dieting, food obsession and body dissatisfaction. When we follow these Strategies daily, we will transform our relationship with food and our bodies, we will create new habits and our body will naturally return to a healthy weight, size and shape.

1. Bite, Chew, Swallow, Wait. This strategy reminds me to enjoy my food and listen to my body. My body is wise and it is now guiding me to the right thoughts and actions that create health and slimness in my body.
2. Leave Some Food on Your Plate. This strategy reminds me that I am in control of what and how much I eat, not the plate, not the restaurant, not other people. I listen to my body, I break habits, I honor my needs.
3. Drink Your Water 6x8. My body is more than 70% water and it needs water to function efficiently. This strategy reminds me to honor my body's needs.
4. Exercise for 20, 3 to 5 days. This strategy reminds me that moving my body leads to vitality, health, stamina and strength. I dedicate myself to find fun and enjoyable ways to stay active.
5. Feed Your Mind, Change What You Say. This strategy reminds me that "what you say is what you get." I dedicate myself to replace all negative, demeaning and hurtful thoughts about myself with supportive, loving and affirmative thoughts.

6. Do Self-Hypnosis Every Day. This strategy helps me to remember that true, lasting change takes place at a deep subconscious level. I use hypnosis to make positive changes without the struggle.

7. Pamper Yourself, Don't Delay. This strategy reminds me to nurture and care for myself in many ways. I know that when I feel joyful and at peace with myself, food automatically loses importance in my life.

To download a full-color list of these strategies to put on your refrigerator or near your desk, go to http://www.donateyourweight.com/images/7strat.pdf

APPENDIX IV

PARTICIPANT FEEDBACK FORM

At Donate Your Weight we value the feedback of our participants and will incorporate your ideas into future products and services. Use the space below to give us your feedback. You can e-mail your feedback to info@donateyourweight.com or you can fax it to (562) 856-1514. Or, if it's more convenient for you, please call our customer comment line and leave your feedback there. Simply call (214) 615-6505 x4921

1. This program is laid out so that it's easy to follow. Yes/No

Please expand on your answer: _____
_____
_____

2. I have lost weight using this program. Yes/No
Tell us what you did to make this program work for you:
_____
_____
_____

3. Using this program resulted in changes besides weight loss. Yes/No Please explain you answer.

_____
_____
_____

4. Use the space below to provide any feedback you have, positive, negative or neutral. Feel free to offer suggestions.

_____

_____

_____

Thank you,
Sheri O. Zampelli, M.S., CCH
Program Developer and Founder of Donate Your Weight

About the Author

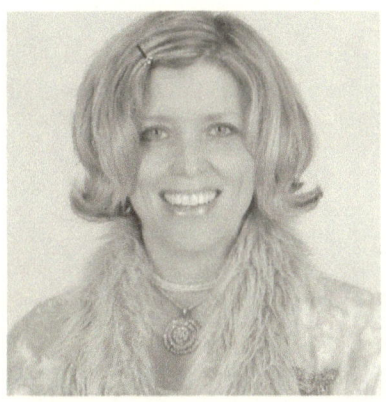

Sheri O. Zampelli, M.S., CCH is the author of *From Sabotage to Success-How to Overcome Self-Defeating Behavior and Reach Your True Potential* and founder of Donate Your Weight. She discovered the power of hypnosis and the Master Mind principle in 1990, after years of struggle with life-threatening addictions, weight and eating struggles, and bouts of extreme depression. Her goal is to share these powerful tools with thousands of people worldwide. Sheri has a master's degree in counseling and teaches topics such as group dynamics and addictive behavior at the college and university level. She works with groups and individuals to help them achieve lifelong goals. For more information, visit www.sherizampelli.com or www.donateyourweight.com

978-0-595-46536-1
0-595-46536-6

www.ingramcontent.com/pod-product-compliance
Lightning Source LLC
Chambersburg PA
CBHW020430290526
45785CB00002B/777